P

SEE PAGE 128 FOR ORDERING INFORMATION

ABBREVIATIONS							
bid	twice per day	h	hour	mEq	milliequiv	PR	by rectum
BP	blood pressure	Hb	hemoglobin	min	minute	prn	as needed
cm	centimeters	HR	heart rate	ml	milliliters	qd	every day
CNS	central nervous sys	ICP	intracranial	mo	month	qid	4 times/day
CSF	cerebrospinal fluid		pressure	NS	normal	SC	subcutaneous
d	day	IM	intramuscular		saline	SD	standard
D_5W	5% dextrose in H_2O	IO	intraosseous	O_2	oxygen		deviation
ET	endotracheal	IV	intravenous	PMN	neutrophil	SL	sublingual
F	French	J	joules	PO	by mouth	tid	3 times/day
g	grams	kg	kilograms	PPV	+pressure	µg	micrograms
		m^2	square meters		ventilation	yo	years old

Tarascon Publishing, Box 1159, Loma Linda, California 92354

Important Caution - Please Read This!

The information in *Pediatric Emergency Pocketbook* is compiled from sources believed to be reliable, and exhaustive efforts have been put forth to make the book as accurate as possible. *However the accuracy and completeness of this work cannot be guaranteed.* Despite our best efforts this book may contain typographical errors and omissions. The *Pediatric Emergency Pocketbook* is intended as a quick and convenient reminder of information you have already learned elsewhere. The contents are to be used as a guide only, and health care professionals should use sound clinical judgment and individualize therapy to each specific patient care situation. This book is not meant to be a replacement for training, experience, continuing medical education, or studying the latest drug prescribing literature. This book is sold without warranties of any kind, express or implied, and the publisher and editors disclaim any liability, loss, or damage caused by the contents. *If you do not wish to be bound by the foregoing cautions & conditions, you may return your undamaged book for a full refund.*

The Tarascon Pediatric Emergency Pocketbook, 3rd Ed

ISBN 1-882742-11-7. Copyright © 1995,1997,1999 Mako Publishing, Inc, Winter Park, Florida. Printed in the USA. All rights reserved. Published & marketed under exclusive license by Tarascon Publishing (Tarascon Inc, Loma Linda, California). No portion of this publication may be reproduced or stored in a retrieval system in any form or by any means (including electronic, mechanical, photocopying, etc.) without prior written permission from us. We welcome suggestions for improving this book. The cover is a detail from the woodcut *"Of a fruitful and well-spoken housewife"*, Francesco Petrarcas, Germany, 1620.

EDITORS		EDITORIAL BOARD
Steven G. Rothrock MD, FACEP, FAAP; Department of Emergency Medicine, Orlando Regional Medical Center, Orlando, FL **Steven M. Green MD**, FACEP; Professor Emerg. Med., EM. Residency Director, Loma Linda University School of Medicine, Loma Linda, CA	**Michael Gerardi MD**, FAAP, FACEP; Vice Chairman, Department of Emergency Medicine, Morristown Memorial Hospital, NJ **Daniel Isaacman MD**, FAAP;Assoc Prof Emerg Med Eastern Virginia Med. School, Director, Peds EM, Children's Hosp. of the King's Daughter	**Larry Mellick MD, FAAP,** FACEP; Professor of Emergency Medicine, Chairman, Medical College Georgia, Augusta, GA **Alfred Sacchetti MD,** FACEP Director of Research Our Lady of Lourdes Hospital, Camden, NJ

Age Based Estimates for Vital Signs and Weight (BP - mean ± 2 standard deviations)

AGE	Weight(kg)	Heart rate	Resp Rate	Systolic BP	Diastolic BP
premature	1	145/min	~40	42 ± 10	21 ± 8
premature	1-2	135	~40	50 ± 10	28 ± 8
newborn	2-3	125	~40	60 ± 10	37 ± 8
1 month	4	120	24-35	80 ± 16	46 ± 16
6 month	7	130	24-35	89 ± 29	60 ± 10
1 year	10	120	20-30	96 ± 30	66 ± 25
2-3 years	12-14	115	20-30	99 ± 25	64 ± 25
4-5 years	16-18	100	20-30	99 ± 20	65 ± 20
6-8 years	20-26	100	12-25	100 ± 15	60 ± 10
10-12 yr	32-42	75	12-25	110 ± 17	60 ± 10
>14 yr	>50	70	12-18	118 ± 20	60 ± 10

Resuscitation Equipment / Drugs Based on Length, Weight, or Age

Length (cm)	58-70	70-85	85-95	95-107	107-124	124-138	138-156
Weight (kg)	5-7	8-11	12-14	15-17	18-24	25-32	33-40
Age (years)	0.5	1	2	3	5	8-10	>12
Bag mask	infant	child	child	child	child	child/adult	adult
Oral airway	infant	small child	child	child	child	small adult	adult
Laryngeal mask	1	2	2	2	2.5	2.5-3	3
Oxygen mask	newborn	peds	peds	peds	adult	adult	adult
ET Tube	3.0/3.5	3.5/4.0	4.0/4.5	4.5	5.0	5.5	6.0
Laryngoscope	1 Miller	1 Miller	2 Miller	2a	2a	2-3a	3a
Suction catheter	8F	8-10F	10F	10F	10F	10F	12F
Stylet	6F	6F	6F	6F	14F	14F	14F
Nasogastric tube	5-8F	8-10F	10F	10-12F	12-14F	14-18F	18F
Urine Catheter	5-8F	8-10F	10F	10-12F	10-12F	12-14F	16F
Chest Tube	10-12F	16-20F	20-24F	20-24F	24-32F	28-32F	32-40F
ampicillin	250-350	400-550	600-700	750-850	900-1200	1250-1600	1650-2000
atropine	0.1-0.14	0.16-.22	0.24-.28	0.3-.34	0.36-.48	0.5-.64	0.66-.80
bicarb (mEq)	5-7	8-11	12-14	15-17	18-24	25-32	33-40
ceftriaxone	250-350	400-550	600-700	750-850	900-1200	1250-1600	1650-2000
cefotaxime	250-350	400-550	600-700	750-850	900-1200	1250-1600	1650-2000
defibrillation (J)	10-14	16-22	24-28	30-34	36-48	50-64	66-80
dextrose (g)	5-7	8-11	12-14	15-17	18-24	25-32	33-40
diazepam	0.5-2.1	0.8-3.3	1.2-4.2	1.5-5.1	1.8-7	2.5-9	3.3-10
epinephrine	0.05-.07	0.08-.11	0.12-.14	0.15-.17	0.18-.24	0.25-.32	0.33-.40
lidocaine	5-7	8-11	12-14	15-17	18-24	25-32	33-40
mannitol (g)	5-7	8-11	12-14	15-17	18-24	25-32	33-40
midazolam	0.5-.7	0.8-1.1	1.2-1.4	1.5-1.7	1.8-2.4	2.5-3.2	3.3-4
normal saline[b]	100-140	160-220	240-280	300-340	360-480	500-640	660-800
succinylcholine	10-14	16-22	24-28	30-34	36-48	50-64	66-80

All drugs are in mg unless otherwise specified. [a]Miller or Macintosh. [b]Bolus (ml) for hypovolemia.

Cardiovascular Drugs: IV Infusions / Mixtures

Drug Solution	1 ml/hr =	Infusion Rate	Drug Preparation
epinephrine (1 mg/ml)	0.1 µg/kg/min	0.1-2.0 µg/kg/min	0.6 mg/kg in D5W in total volume of 100 ml
isoproterenol (1 mg/5 ml)	0.1 µg/kg/min	0.1-1.0 µg/kg/min	0.6 mg/kg in D5W in total volume of 100 ml
norepinephrine (1 mg/ml)	0.1 µg/kg/min	0.1-1.0 µg/kg/min	0.6 mg/kg in D5W in total volume of 100 ml
dopamine (40 mg/ml)	1.0 µg/kg/min	2.0-20 µg/kg/min	6.0 mg/kg in D5W in total volume of 100 ml
dobutamine (250 mg vial)	1.0 µg/kg/min	5.0-20 µg/kg/min	6.0 mg/kg in D5W in total volume of 100 ml
lidocaine 2% (20 mg/ml)	20 µg/min	20-50 µg/kg/min	300 mg in D5W in total volume of 250 ml
phenylephrine (10 mg/ml)	1.33 µg/min	0.5-5 µg/kg/min	20 mg in D5W in total volume of 250 ml
procainamide (100 mg/ml)	20 µg/min	20-80 µg/kg/min	300 mg in D5W in total volume of 250 ml

CPR Maneuvers and Techniques In Newborns, Infants, & Children

Maneuver	Newborn	Infant(<1 year)	Child (1-8 years)
Open Airway	Slightly extend neck Use shoulder roll to maintain neutral position	Head tilt or chin lift (unless trauma then jaw lift)	Head tilt or chin lift (unless trauma then jaw lift)
Breathing *Initial*	May require 30-40 cm H2O pressure	Two breaths at 1-1.5 sec/breath	Two breaths at 1-1.5 sec/breath
Subsequent	40-60 breaths/min at lower pressure	20 breaths/min	20 breaths/min
Circulation *Check pulse*	Brachial	Brachial or femoral	Carotid
Compress if	Heart rate < 60, or 60-80 and not increasing despite ventilation with 100% oxygen for at least 30 seconds		
Compress area	Chest/midsternum	Lower 1/3 sternum	Lower 1/3 sternum
Compress with	Two thumbs encircle chest or two fingers	Two or three fingers	Heel of one hand
Depth	1/2 - 3/4 inch	1/2 - 1 inch	1 - 1 1/2 inches
Rate	120/min	at least 100/min	100/min
Ratio	3:1 (interpose breaths)	5:1 (interpose breaths)	5:1 (interpose breaths)
Airway Obstruction	Back blows Chest thrusts	Back blows Chest thrusts	Abdominal thrusts

Pediatric Bradycardia

- Assess ABC's
- Secure airway
- Administer 100% oxygen
- Assess vital signs
- Start IV or intraosseous line

↓

| NO | ← | Severe cardiopulmonary compromise?
(poor perfusion, ↓BP, or respiratory difficulty) | → | YES |

↓ (NO)

- Observe
- Support ABC's
- Consider transfer to advanced life support facility

↓ (YES)

Perform chest compressions if (despite oxygenation and ventilation):
- Heart rate < 80 and age < 2 years
- Heart rate < 60 and age > 2 years
(Hypothermia may require protocol deviation)

↓

Epinephrine
- IV/IO: 0.01 mg/kg of 1:10,000
- Endotracheal: 0.1 mg/kg of 1:1,000
- Repeat q3-5 minutes at same dose

↓

Atropine
- 0.02 mg/kg IV/IO/ET
- Minimum dose 0.1 mg, and maximum 0.5 mg for child and 1 mg for adolescent
- May be repeated once

↓

- Consider external or esophageal pacing
- Consider digoxin Fab fragments if digoxin toxicity
- Consider glucagon if toxicity from β-blockers or calcium channel blockers

Pediatric Cardiac Arrest

Determine pulselessness and begin CPR
Confirm cardiac rhythm in more than one lead

Ventricular fibrillation or pulseless V-tachycardia	Asystole	Pulseless electrical activity (PEA, EMD)

Ventricular fibrillation or pulseless V-tachycardia

- Continue CPR
- Secure airway
- Hyperventilate with 100% O_2
- IV/IO (no delay in defibrillation)

- Defibrillate up to 3 times if needed, 2 J/kg, 4 J/kg, 4 J/kg

Epinephrine (*first dose*)
- IV/IO: 0.01 mg/kg of 1:10,000
- Endotracheal: 0.1 mg/kg of 1:1,000

- Defibrillate 4 J/kg 30-60 seconds after each med dose

- Lidocaine 1 mg/kg IV/IO

- Defibrillate 4 J/kg 30-60 seconds after each med dose

- Epinephrine (*subsequent doses*): 0.1-0.2 mg/kg IV/IO/ET of 1:1000, repeat q3-5 minutes
- Lidocaine 1 mg/kg
- Consider bretylium 5 mg/kg IV then 10 mg/kg

Asystole

Pulseless electrical activity (PEA, EMD)

Identify and treat causes
- Severe hypoxemia
- Severe acidosis
- Severe hypovolemia
- Tension pneumothorax
- Cardiac tamponade
- Profound hypothermia

- CPR, secure airway
- Hyperventilate with 100% O_2
- IV or IO access

Epinephrine (*first dose*)
- IV/IO: 0.01 mg/kg of 1:10,000
- Endotracheal: 0.1 mg/kg of 1:1,000

Epinephrine (*subsequent doses*):
- 0.1-0.2 mg/kg IV/IO/ET of 1:1000
- repeat q3-5 minutes

Neonatal Resuscitation

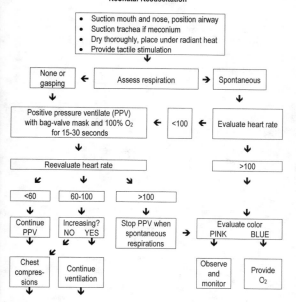

- Suction mouth and nose, position airway
- Suction trachea if meconium
- Dry thoroughly, place under radiant heat
- Provide tactile stimulation

None or gasping ← Assess respiration → Spontaneous

Positive pressure ventilate (PPV) with bag-valve mask and 100% O_2 for 15-30 seconds ← <100 ← Evaluate heart rate

Reevaluate heart rate

>100

<60   60-100   >100

Continue PPV   Increasing? NO YES   Stop PPV when spontaneous respirations → Evaluate color PINK   BLUE

Chest compressions   Continue ventilation   Observe and monitor   Provide O_2

Initiate drug therapy if heart rate remains <80 after 30 seconds of PPV with 100% O_2 and chest compressions

O_2 is not needed for peripheral cyanosis. Check heart rate every 30 sec. Pulse oximetry is accurate in newborns if saturation is >40% and is not affected by fetal hemoglobin. By 5 min., vaginally delivered neonates have rapid rise of O_2 saturation to 80% on room air.

Apgar Scoring

Sign	0	1	2
Heart rate	absent	<100	>100
Respiratory effort	absent	slow / irregular	good, cry
Muscle tone	flaccid	some extremity flexion	active motion
Reflex irritability	no response	grimace	vigorous cry
Color	pale	cyanotic	completely pink

Normal Neonatal Blood Pressure for Different Birth Weights

Weight	<1 kg	1-2 kg	2-3 kg	>3 kg
Systolic BP	40-60	50-60	50-70	50-80
Diastolic BP	15-35	20-40	25-45	30-50

A respiratory rate of 60 to 90 is normal in the first few hours of life. A 5-minute Apgar score $\leq$ 3 predicts poor neurologic outcome.

Treatable causes of neonatal distress: respiratory insufficiency, hypoglycemia, hypocalcemia (usually does not occur until 24-48 hours), hypothermia, blood loss. *Treatment of neonatal distress*: (1) See algorithm on page 7. (2) Administer O_2 if central cyanosis and heart rate $\leq$ 100. (3) Ventilate with bag-valve-mask (BVM) if apneic, or respirations insufficient to keep heart rate >100. (4) Place orogastric tube if BVM over 2 minutes. Use #8 French feeding tube and a 20 ml syringe (length = ear lobe to nose distance or earlobe to xiphoid distance in cm). The tube must be put in through mouth and not the nose because neonates are obligate nose breathers. (5) Intubation is indicated if ineffective respirations with BVM, BVM >2 min, diaphragmatic hernia, or meconium aspiration requiring tracheal suctioning.

Size of Endotracheal Tube and Laryngoscope Blade

Gestational age	Birth weight (g)	Size of ET Tube[1]	Blade size
<28 weeks	<1,000	2.5	Number 0 Miller
28-34 weeks	1,000-2,000	2.5-3.0	Number 0 Miller
34-38 weeks	2,000-3,000	3.0-3.5	Number 0 Miller
>38 weeks	Term (>3,000)	3.5-4.0	Number 1 Miller

[1]*Internal diameter in millimeters*

Airway and resuscitation tips: Once ET tube is secured, shorten the ET tube so that only 4 cm protrude from mouth to decrease dead space and limit tube kinking. Never use more than 100 mmHg to suction. During intubation a blade sweep of tongue should be avoided and blade should just be placed over tongue.

Chest compressions: Perform chest compressions if after 15-30 seconds of assisted ventilation the heart rate is <60 or 60-80 and not increasing. Compress ½ to ¾ inches at 120/minute while ventilating 40-60 breaths/min. Treat pneumothorax by placing 22 gauge IV catheter in the 4th intercostal space at the anterior axillary line. Then place a #10F chest tube if < 1500g or #12 if ≥ 1500 g.

Drug therapy: Indicated if asystole or if HR<80 despite adequate ventilation and chest compressions for 30 seconds. Atropine is of limited value in the acute phase of neonatal resuscitation.

- *Epinephrine*: If HR <80 after 30 seconds of CPR. Dose 0.01-0.03 mg/kg IV (0.1-0.3 ml/kg of 1:10,000) with ET dose 10 times higher. Repeat q5 min prn.
- *Volume expanders*: Administer if signs of hypovolemia (pallor, weak pulses with normal HR, poor response to resuscitation, poor capillary refill, and/or low blood pressure). Use whole blood cross-matched to mother, 5% albumin, or other colloids/crystalloids. Treat with 10-20 ml/kg IV over 5-10 min.
- *Sodium bicarbonate*: 2 mEq/kg IV of *4.2% solution* over 2 minutes. Rapid administration may cause venous irritation or provoke intracranial bleeding.
- *Dopamine*: Consider if blood pressure fails to respond to other therapies.
- *Naloxone*: Administer 0.1 mg/kg IV if severe respiratory depression and maternal narcotic administration in the prior 4 hours. Use of naloxone in neonate is controversial and some recommend avoiding this agent, as it may precipitate seizures if mother used narcotics chronically.
- *Glucose*: Hypoglycemia is most common in premature or small for gestational age infants following a prolonged and difficult labor, mothers on ritodrine or terbutaline, and infants of diabetics. Hypoxia, hypothermia, hyperthermia and sepsis also deplete glucose stores. Treat with 1-2 ml/kg of $D_{10}W$ IV push, then infuse 6-8 mg/kg/min.

Abnormal Glucose for Neonates

Administer glucose to all neonates with bedside glucose <50 mg/dl, as this test may be inaccurate below this level.

Age	Hypoglycemia
premature	<25
full term <72h	<35
full term >72h	<45

Vascular Access

Central Venous Catheter Diameter Based on Age and Catheter Site (internal diameter-French [F])	Age (years)	Internal jugular vein	Subclavian vein	Femoral vein
	0 - 0.5	3 F	3 F	3 F
	0.5 - 2	3 F	3 F	3 - 4 F
	3 - 6	4 F	4 F	4 F
	7 - 12	4 – 5 F	4 - 5 F	4 - 5 F

Central Venous Catheter Depth Based on Age, Weight, and Catheter Site

Age	Weight (kg)	Height (cm)	Internal Jugular Vein	Subclavian Vein	Femoral Vein
1 month	4.2	55	6.0 cm	5.5 cm	15.7 cm
6 months	7.8	68	7.3 cm	6.6 cm	19.1 cm
1 year	10.2	76	8.0 cm	7.3 cm	21.1 cm
2 years	12.8	88	9.2 cm	8.3 cm	24.2 cm
4 years	16.5	103	10.6 cm	9.6 cm	28.1 cm
6 years	20.5	116	11.8 cm	10.7 cm	31.4 cm
8 years	26	127	12.9 cm	11.7 cm	34.2 cm
10 years	31	137	13.8 cm	12.5 cm	36.8 cm
14 years	50	165	16.5 cm	14.9 cm	44 cm

Umbilical Artery/Vein Catheterization

Umbilical vein is a single thin walled vessel in umbilical cord that is preferred for vascular access during neonatal resuscitation. The two thick walled arteries may also be used. To catheterize umbilical vein, follow the listed steps:

- Prepare the abdomen and cord in sterile fashion, loosely tie umbilical tape to cord base for anchoring & hemostasis, & cut cord with scalpel 2 cm from abdominal wall.
- Locate vein and remove any visible clot, flush catheter with heparin solution.
- Use 3.5-4 French (Fr) catheter if < 2 kg and 5-8 Fr for > 2 kg neonates.
- Advance umbilical catheter(5-8 Fr) through vein until blood return or 4-5 cm.
- Shoulder (lateral clavicle) - umbilicus length X 0.6 places tip above diaphragm.
- Tighten umbilical tape to secure, and withdraw after resuscitation.
- Umbilical artery (UA) catheterization: after dilating with iris forcep, insert tip of catheter to lumen. Estimated depth of low UA catheter: [Birth weight (kg) + 7] cm.

Intraosseous (IO)

Place IO in proximal tibia (1-2 cm distal + medial to tuberosity), distal tibia (medial malleolus - tibial shaft junction), or distal femur (as condyle tapers into shaft). After local anesthetic, and site prepared in sterile manner, puncture skin, direct needle away from growth plate. Push + rotate gently until "pop" with trap door like effect and advance 0.5-1 cm. Aspirate for labs(Hb, type & cross) + and infuse with large syringe. Any drug or blood can be given IO. Watch for leak.

Airway Management

	Age	Weight (kg)	ET Tube[1]	Laryngoscope
Endotracheal Tube and Blade Size	premature	1.5	2.5 - 3.0	Miller 0
	term	3.0	3.0 - 3.5	Miller 0-1
	3 months	5.5	3.5 - 4.0	Miller 1
	6 months	7	4.0	Miller 1
	1 year	10	4.5	Miller 1
	2 years	12	4.5	Miller 1
	3 years	14	5.0	Miller/Macintosh 2
	4 years	16	5.5	Miller/Macintosh 2
	5 years	18	5.5	Miller/Macintosh 2
	6-7 years	20-22	6.0	Miller/Macintosh 2
	8-10 years	25-30	6.0 - 6.5	Miller/Macintosh 2
	10-12 years	30-35	6.5	Miller/Macintosh 2
	12-14 years	35-40	7.0	Miller/Macintosh 3

[1]Internal diameter in millimeters

Formula for estimating ET tube size based on age
- Tube internal diameter estimate (mm) = [16 + age in years] ÷ 4
- Use uncuffed ET tubes under age 8.
- If cuffed subtract 0.5 mm from size estimate.
- see page 3 for age, length and weight based estimation for ET tube and meds.

Anatomic Indicators of Difficult Pediatric Airway
- *Oropharyngeal exam* - inability to visualize tonsillar pillars, soft palate, or uvula
- *Atlanto-occipital joint* - extension less than 35 degrees
- *Thyromental distance* - distance of > 2 adult fingerwidths (3 cm) from the mandibular ramus to the thyroid cartilage in an adolescent or child **Or** more than 1 adult fingerwidth (1.5 cm) in an infant. Measure with neck in neutral position.
- *Temporomandibular joint* - limited hinge movement of temporomandibular joint (e.g. juvenile rheumatoid arthritis, scoliosis, inflammatory trismus from deep space infection, or mandibular fracture)
- *Congenital airway anomalies* - cleft palate, maxillary or mandibular anomalies, micrognathia, macroglossia, glossoptosis.
- *Maxillary abnormality* - protruding maxillary incisors or maxillofacial trauma
- *Upper airway swelling/obstruction* - bleeding, infection, burn, or inhalation injury

Steps for Rapid Sequence Intubation

Equipment
- ready 2 wall suction devices with Yankauer tips, check laryngoscope lights
- appropriate size ET tube and back-up 0.5 to 1 size smaller, consider stylet
- check integrity of inflatable cuff, if present (no cuff if ≤ 8 years of age)

Patient Preparation
- raise bed to comfortable height (e.g., patient's nose at intubator's xiphoid)
- prepare alternate airway plan: transtracheal jet ventilation, cricothyrotomy (>8y)
- estimate patient's weight (e.g., Broeslow tape)
- confirm working pulse oximeter and cardiac monitor
- specify personnel for (1) cricoid pressure, (2) neck immobilization if trauma, (3) handling ET tube, (4) watching O_2 sat & cardiac monitors, and (5) medications
- position head appropriately (sniffing position if no trauma)
- draw up all drugs in syringes and ensure secure IV access is available
- preoxygenate with 100% oxygen for at least 3-4 minutes (if time permits)
- perform Sellick maneuver (cricoid pressure)

Medication
- lidocaine 1.5 mg/kg IV if head injured (to attenuate rise in intracranial pressure)
- atropine 0.02 mg/kg IV (minimum dose 0.1 mg) if < 5 years
- consider use of defasciculating agent IV (then wait 1.5 to 2 minutes)
- administer sedating and paralyzing agent IV

Drugs for Rapid Sequence Intubation

Agent	Dose IV (mg/kg)	Onset (min)	Key Properties
Defasciculating drug[1]			may occasionally cause paralysis
pancuronium	0.01	3	histamine release, tachycardia
rocuronium	0.06	2-3	
succinylcholine	0.1	3	fasciculations, ↑ BP,ICP,GI,eye pressure
vecuronium	0.01	3	minimal tachycardia
Sedating drug			
etomidate	0.3-0.4	1-2	minimal blood pressure effect
fentanyl	2-10 µg/kg	1-2	↑ ICP, chest wall rigidity
ketamine	1-2	< 1	↑ BP, ↑ ICP, ↑ GI and eye pressure
midazolam	0.1-0.2	1-3	hypotension
propofol	1.0-2.5	< 1	hypotension
thiopental	2-5	< 1	hypotension, bronchospasm
Paralyzing drug			
Succinylcholine[2]	1-2	<1	fasciculations ↑BP,ICP,GI,eye pressures
pancuronium	0.1	1-5	tachycardia, prolonged action
rocuronium	0.6-1.2	0.5-1.5	rapid onset, short duration (25-60 min)
vecuronium	0.1 - 0.3	1-4	prolonged action

[1]Unnecessary <5 years. [2]Use 2 mg/kg if <10 kg, & 1.5 mg/kg if defasciculating agent used.

Steps to Perform after Intubation	• Check tube placement (breath sounds, CO_2 detector) • Inflate cuff (if present) then release cricoid pressure • Measure and record tube depth (see below) • Reassess patient's clinical status • Obtain CXR to verify correct placement depth • Consider longer-acting sedative and paralytics

Formulas for Estimating depth of ET tube after intubation

- Distance in cm from midtrachea to incisors/gum line = 3 x (ET tube ID[1])
- Distance in cm from midtrachea to incisors/gum line = 12 + (age in years)/2
- Distance in cm from midtrachea to incisors/gum line = (height in cm)/10 + 5
- Distance in cm from midtrachea to nares (for nasotracheal) = 12 + (age in yrs)/2

[1]ID - internal diameter in mm

Laryngeal Mask Airway Sizes if Intubation Unsuccessful

Mask Size	Patient weight	Internal diameter (mm)	cuff volume (ml)
1	< 6.5 kg	5.25	2 - 5
2	6.5 - 20 kg	7	7 - 10
2.5	20 - 30 kg	8.4	14
3	30 - 70 kg	10	15 - 20
4	70 - 90 kg	12	25 - 30
5	> 90 kg	11.5	30 - 40

Rescue Procedure for Transtracheal Jet Ventilation

Place a 14-gauge IV catheter attached to 5ml syringe through cricothyroid membrane. Remove needle, leaving catheter and confirm placement by aspirating air. Attach 3.0 mm ET tube adapter to IV catheter, or attach 3 ml locking syringe (without plunger) to 3 mm ET tube adapter. Attach 10-50 psi 100% O_2 source and deliver O_2 at 20 bursts/minute with inspiratory to expiratory ratio of 1:2 or 1:3.

	Age	Initial PSI	Tidal Volume (ml)
Parameters for transtracheal jet ventilation	< 5 years	5	100
	5-8 years	5-10	240-340
	8-12 years	10-25	340-625
	> 12 years	30-50	700-1000

Guidelines for Initiating Mechanical Ventilation

Item	Neonates & Infants	Older Children
Ventilator	pressure-limited if weight <10 kg	volume-limited
Resp Rate	30-40 per minute	normal for age
I:E ratio[1]	1:2	1:2
Setting	Begin peak inspiratory pressure at 16 mmHg, ↑ 2 mm Hg until good excursion	tidal volume 10-12 ml/kg
PEEP[2]	start at 3-4 cm H_2O	start at 3-4 cm H_2O
FiO_2	5-10% above preintubation FiO_2, adjust to oxygen saturation	

[1]Inspiratory/expiratory ratio, which varies with higher respiratory rate and specific diseases.
[2]Peak end expiratory pressure.

Analgesia and Sedation

Agent Trade name	Dose (mg/kg)	Route	Onset (min)	Duration (hours)	Comments
chloral hydrate	50-75	PO/PR	30	3-4	GI irritant, rare cardiac arrhythmias, possible carcinogen
diazepam *Valium*	0.1 0.5	IV PR	< 1	1-2	↓respirations, ↓BP
fentanyl *Sublimaze*	2-3 µg/kg	IV	2	0.5	↓respirations, ↓BP, bradycardia, rare chest wall rigidity
flumazenil *Romazicon*	0.01- 0.03	IV	< 1	1	reverses benzodiazepines (e.g. lorazepam, midazolam, diazepam)
ketamine *Ketalar*	1-2 4 5-10	IV IM PO	< 1 5 30	0.25 0.5-1.0 1-2	↑BP, ↑intracranial/ocular pressure, rare laryngospasm, co-administer atropine .01 mg/kg to ↓salivation
meperidine *Demerol*	1 1-2	IV IM	< 1 0.25	0.5-1.0 2-3	↓respirations, ↓BP, anticholinergic properties
methohexital *Brevital*	20	PR	15	0.5	↓respirations, ↓BP
midazolam *Versed*	0.15 0.15 0.2-0.3	IV IM PR	2 10-15 10-15	0.5 0.75 1	↓respirations, ↓BP (can also begin orally at 0.7 mg/kg: onset 10-15 min, duration 1 h)
morphine	0.1	IV	< 5	3-4	↓respirations, ↓BP
naloxone *Narcan*	0.1	IV, IM, SC	< 1	< 1	reverses narcotics (e.g. morphine, demerol)
nitrous oxide	30%	inhaled	1-2	<5	patient holds mask to self-titrate

Oral Analgesic Agents

Agent	Dose (mg/kg)	Frequency	Concentration / Comments
acetaminophen	15	q4h	80 mg/0.8 ml (dropper) or 160 mg per 5 ml
acetaminophen with codeine	0.5 to 1	q4h	acetaminophen 120 mg + codeine 12 mg per 5 ml (dose in mg/kg based on codeine)
aspirin	10-15	q4h	no elixir available
hydrocodone[1] (*Lortab* elixir)	-	q4-6h	Dose: > 12 years – 10 ml q 4-6 hours Dose: 6 - 12 years – 5 ml q 4-6 hours
ibuprofen	5-10	q4-8h	*Children's Motrin*: 100 mg per 5 ml
meperidine[1]	1-2	q4h	50 mg per 5 ml
naproxen[1]	5-7	q8h	125 mg per 5 ml

[1]only approved for select ages/indications, consult manufacturer's product labeling.

Anaphylaxis

Anaphylaxis Treatment

Drug	Dose -mg/kg	Route	Indications
epinephrine	0.01	SC/IM	mild to moderate symptoms
	infusion[1]	IV	airway compromise, severe hypotension administer 0.1 ml/kg (10 µg/kg) of 1:10,000 solution IV over 2 minutes
Solu-Medrol	2	IV	moderate/severe symptoms
Benadryl	1	IV/IM	moderate/severe symptoms
cimetidine	5	IV/IM	if no resp. symptoms (bronchoconstricts)
glucagon	0.03-0.1	IV/SC	if patient taking a β-blocker
albuterol	2.5-5 mg	nebulized	bronchospasm
epinephrine	0.25-.5 ml	nebulized	Stridor, use 2.25% solution

[1]*Epinephrine infusion*: see page 4. Use caution, as lethal complications can occur.
Bee Sting Remove stinger, rinse, apply ice. 0.005 ml/kg epi locally if not end-organ site.

Apparent Life Threatening Events (ALTE)

Apnea – cessation of breathing for > 20 seconds or shorter cessation associated with bradycardia, pallor, or cyanosis.
ALTE – apnea associated with color change (cyanosis or plethora), a loss of muscle tone, and choking or gagging. (formerly known as near SIDS).

Evaluation and Management

- ADMIT all with true ALTE episode
- Immediately apply cardiac monitor, check O_2 saturation and glucose
- Obtain the following on all patients – CBC, electrolytes, ECG, CXR.
- Consider additional tests based on history and examination – spinal tap, urinalysis, EEG, barium swallow, cranial CT, nasopharyngeal swab for RSV and pertussis, Echocardiogram, Holter monitor, sleep studies.

Etiologies of Apnea in Infancy

- *Infection* – central nervous system or sepsis, or respiratory infection
- *Central nervous system disease* – seizures, hemorrhage, ↑ pressure, central hypoventilation
- *GI* – reflux, tracheoesophageal fistula, swallowing disorder
- *Pulmonary* – edema, bleed, hypoplastic lung, respiratory distress syndrome
- *Cardiac* – congenital heart disease, shock, dysrhythmia, ↑ QT
- *Metabolic* – ↓glucose, ↓Ca^{+2}, ↓Na^{+2}, inborn metabolic errors
- *Musculoskeletal* – infant botulism, Guillain Barre, congenital myopathies
- *Other* – anemia, poisons, hypothermia, hyperthermia, child abuse
- *Airway obstruction* - multiple diseases

Burns and Burn Therapy

Fluid resuscitation in burn victims

Parkland formula	• Lactated ringers 4 ml/kg/% burn BSA[1] in 1st 24 h + maintenance fluid, with ½ over 1st 8 hours, and ½ over subsequent 16 h
Alternatives (See page 38 for maintenance fluid rate)	• *Amended Parkland formula*: for ED stays < 8 hours. IV rate over maintenance[2] (ml/h) = [weight(kg) X burn BSA%] ÷ 4 • *Carvajal's formula*: Carvajal' solution 5,000 ml/m² of burn + maintenance 2000 ml/m² in 1st 24h , with ½ over the 1st 8h and ½ over the subsequent 16h.

[1]BSA = body surface area.

Estimation of Burn Surface Area

Age in Years	<1	1	5	10	15
head	19%	17%	13%	11%	9%
neck	2	2	2	2	2
half of trunk(ant or post)	13	13	13	13	13
one buttock	2.5	2.5	2.5	2.5	2.5
genitalia	1	1	1	1	1
upper (3) or lower (4) arm	3-4	3-4	3-4	3-4	3-4
one hand (2.5) or foot (3.5)	2.5-3.5	2.5-3.5	2.5-3.5	2.5-3.5	2.5-3.5
one thigh	5	6.5	8.5	9	9.5
one leg (below knee)	5	5	5.5	6	6.5

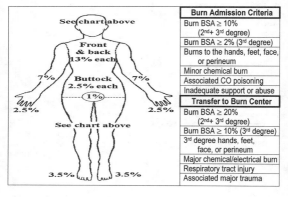

Burn Admission Criteria
Burn BSA ≥ 10% (2nd+ 3rd degree)
Burn BSA ≥ 2% (3rd degree)
Burns to the hands, feet, face, or perineum
Minor chemical burn
Associated CO poisoning
Inadequate support or abuse

Transfer to Burn Center
Burn BSA ≥ 20% (2nd+ 3rd degree)
Burn BSA ≥ 10% (3rd degree)
3rd degree hands, feet, face, or perineum
Major chemical/electrical burn
Respiratory tract injury
Associated major trauma

Figure labels: See chart above; Front & back 13% each; 7%; 7%; Buttock 2.5% each; 1%; 2.5%; 2.5%; See chart above; 3.5%; 3.5%

Cardiac Disorders

Normal ECG Values

Age	P-R interval[1]	QRS interval[1]	QRS axis (mean)	QTc[2]
0-7 days	0.08-0.12	0.04-0.08	80-160 (125)	0.34-0.54
1-4 weeks	0.08-0.12	0.04-0.07	60-160 (110)	0.30-0.50
1-3 months	0.08-0.12	0.04-0.08	40-120 (80)	0.32-0.47
3-6 months	0.08-0.12	0.04-0.08	20-80 (65)	0.35-0.46
6-12 months	0.09-0.13	0.04-0.08	0-100 (65)	0.31-0.49
1-3 years	0.10-0.14	0.04-0.08	20-100 (55)	0.34-0.49
3-8 years	0.11-0.16	0.05-0.09	40-80 (60)	< 0.45
8-16 years	0.12-0.17	0.05-0.09	20-80 (65)	< 0.45

[1]seconds [2]QTc = QT interval / (square root of RR interval)

ECG Diagnosis of Chamber Enlargement (Hypertrophy)

Right ventricular hypertrophy/RVH	Biventricular hypertrophy
• R in V1 > 20 mm (> 25 mm < 1 mo) • S in V6 > 6 mm (> 12 mm < 1 mo) • Upright T in V3R, R in V1 after 5 day • QR pattern in V3R, V1	• RVH and (S in V1 or R in V6) exceeding mean for age • LVH and (R in V1 or S in V6) exceeding mean for age
Left ventricular hypertrophy/LVH	**Right atrial hypertrophy**
• R in V6 > 25 mm (> 21 mm < 1 yr) • S in V1 > 30 mm (> 20 mm < 1 yr) • R in V6 + S in V1 > 60 mm (use V5 if R in V5 > R in V6) • Abnormal R/S ratio • S in V1 > 2 X R in V5	• peak P value > 3 mm (< 6 months), > 2.5 mm (≥ 6 months)
	Left atrial hypertrophy
	• P in II > 0.09 seconds • P in V1 with late negative deflection > 0.04 seconds and > 1 mm deep

Chest Pain and Syncope

Cardiac Causes of Chest Pain in Children

• Ischemia from coronary arteritis (e.g. Kawasaki's), coronary artery anomalies, hypertension, hypoxia • Structural anomalies (e.g. aortic stenosis), pulmonic stenosis, idiopathic subaortic stenosis (IHSS)	• Arrhythmias (bradycardia or tachycardia) • ↓ BP with ↓ coronary perfusion • Infectious or inflammatory disease (e.g. pericarditis, myocarditis, endocarditis)

Chest Pain Etiologies Presenting to a Pediatric Emergency Department	Musculoskeletal	25%	Psychogenic	9%
	Respiratory	21%	Trauma	5%
	Idiopathic	21%	GI	4%
	Miscellaneous	11%	Cardiac	4%

Pediatrics 1988;82:319

Syncope Etiologies Presenting to a Pediatric Emergency Department	Vasovagal	50%	Head trauma	5%
	Orthostasis	20%	Migraine	5%
	Atypical seizure	7%	Miscellaneous	13%

Pediatr Emerg Care 1989; 5:80-82

Features Associated with Life Threatening Cause of Syncope

- Family history of cardiomyopathy or sudden death (IHSS, prolonged QT)
- Syncope during exercise or while supine (IHSS, aortic+ pulmonic stenosis, pulmonary hypertension)
- Syncope with chest pain (IHSS, ischemia aortic stenosis)
- Abnormal ECG
- Recurrent syncope
- Fall directly onto face (rapid onset)
- Congenital heart disease
- Drugs with cardiac effects
- Marfanoid appearance or collagen vascular disease in family

Differential Diagnosis of Cyanosis

Detectable cyanosis requires 5g Hb/100 ml of desaturated blood. pO_2 in a right to left "cyanotic" cardiac shunt will not exceed 50 mmHg after 100% O_2 for 10 minutes.

- *Central Cyanosis*: hemoglobinopathies (e.g., methemoglobin, sulfhemoglobin, carboxyhemoglobin), or oxygen desaturation due to impaired lung function, hypoventilation or anatomic shunts (e.g., congenital heart disease)
- *Peripheral cyanosis*: reduced cardiac output, shock, cold exposure, redistribution of blood flow from extremities, arterial or venous obstruction.

"Tet Spells" (Hypercyanotic Spells)

Acute right to left shunting leads to tachypnea, worsened cyanosis, diminished murmur, stroke or death. Precipitants: crying, defecating, exercise, ↓ systemic vascular resistance (SVR), ↓ LV pressure, and RV outflow spasm.

Treatment of "Tet Spells"

- Oxygen – 100%
- Knee chest position or squatting to decrease venous return to heart
- Morphine 0.1 mg/kg - ↓ outflow spasm
- Propanolol[1] 0.025 mg/kg IV to ↓ outflow spasm (cautiously titrate up to 0.1mg/kg)
- NaHCO₃ 1 mEq/kg IV to normalize pH
- NS 20 ml/kg IV to ↓ shunting
- Phenylephrine (2-5 µg/kg/min) – goal is to ↑systolic BP 20% causing ↑SVR.
- Prostaglandin E₁ (0.05-0.2 µg/kg/min) to reopen ductus arteriosis.[2]

[1]May substitute esmolol – see page 57.

[2]Also consider use in sudden cardiovascular collapse/shock in neonate.

Dysrhythmias

Prolonged QT interval: (1) inherited form may be associated with deafness, or (2) acquired due to class I antiarrhythmics (e.g., quinidine, procainamide), amiodarone, phenothiazines, lithium, cyclic antidepressants, $\downarrow K^+$, $\downarrow Ca^{+2}$, $\downarrow Mg^{+2}$, myocarditis, liver disease, weight loss. Children with prolonged QTc may present with syncope or seizures. Treat by correcting disorder or discontinuing drug. QTc = QT interval / (square root of RR interval). See page 17 for age-based normal QTc intervals.

Supraventricular tachycardia (SVT) is due to reentry-bypass tract in 50%, reentry without bypass in 25%, and an ectopic focus with abnormal automaticity in 25%. Children < 4 months old with SVT are more likely to have CHF.

Unstable SVT Management (See page 20)

- Synchronized cardioversion at 0.5 joules/kg, $\uparrow$ to 1 then 2 j/kg if unsuccessful
- Pretreat with lidocaine (1 mg/kg IV) if patient is taking digoxin

Stable SVT Management Options (See page 20)

- Vagal maneuvers (e.g., carotid massage, Valsalva, a bag of ice on face) OR
- Adenosine 0.05 mg/kg IV double each subsequent dose (max 0.25 mg/kg), OR
- Verapamil 0.075-0.15 mg/kg IV (contraindicated if ≤ 1 year old) OR
- Procainamide 50 mg/min or slower IV up to 5-10 mg/kg (stop if wide complex, rhythm converts, or hypotension), then 20-80 µg/kg/minute OR
- β-blocker (contraindicated if severe CHF, asthma, wide complex), OR
- Digoxin (for dose see page 20)

Ventricular tachycardia is generally >120 beats/minute. Aberrant SVT is rare in children. Try lidocaine 1 mg/kg bolus, then infusion 20-40 µg/kg/minute, or procainamide 5-10 mg/kg IV over 30 minutes (see precautions under SVT).

Atrial flutter - atrial rate of ~300 beats/minute. In infants, AF can occur without typical sawtooth pattern or flutter waves. 93% have structural heart disease.

Physiologic Murmurs[1]

Murmur	Age	Location	Timing	Cause
Still's	3-6 y	apex	systole	turbulent LV outflow
pulm ejection	8-14 y	2nd left ICS	systole	RV outflow tract turbulence
supraclavicular	4-14 y	above clavicle	systole	brachiocephalic branching
venous hum[2]	3-6 y	base of neck	entire	venous return
straight back pectus	all	apex		RV filling with inspiration
hemic exertion	all	apex, left ICS	systole	rapid LV ejection
neonatal pulm ejection	<6 months	right 2nd ICS	systole	underdeveloped pulmonary arteries

[1] LV=left ventricle, RV=right ventricle, ICS=intercostal space. Most physiologic murmurs are systolic and are louder with increased cardiac output.
[2] Venous hums decrease with supine position, turning head, and expiration.

Murmur evaluation: Murmurs should be of extra concern if the patient has congenital heart disease, failure to thrive, frequent infections, asthma, chest pain, or syncope. Congenital heart disease is suggested if *one* major or *two* minor criteria:

- *Major*: grade ≥ 3, pansystolic, late systolic, diastolic, CHF, cyanosis.
- *Minor*: grade < 3, systolic, or abnormal CXR, EKG, BP, or S_2 heart sound.

Age-Related Digoxin Dosing

Age	Total digitalizing dose	Maintenance(IV)
premature neonate	20 µg/kg	4 µg/kg/24 hours
term neonate	30 µg/kg	4-5 µg/kg/12 hours
1-24 months	40 µg/kg	5-10 µg/kg/12 hours
2-10 years	35 µg/kg (max 2 mg)	5-10 µg/kg/12h (max 0.125 mg)

Total digitalizing dose (TDD) is given over 16-24 hours: ½ of dose initially IV, followed by ¼ dose at both 8 and 16 hours. Oral doses are 20% greater, with maintenance dose 12.5% of TDD q12h starting 12h after TDD complete. Always have 2 persons independently calculate and verify any dose of digoxin. Closely monitor potassium to avoid hypokalemia, which can exacerbate digoxin toxicity.

Supraventricular Tachycardia Management

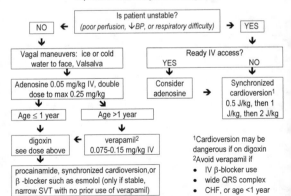

Neonatal Rashes

Transient benign vascular phenomena occurring in neonates (1) *acrocyanosis* - blue, purple discoloration due to cold stress, (2) *cutis marmorata* - reticulated cyanosis or marbling of skin symmetrically involving the trunk and extremities, (3) *harlequin color change* - when infant lies horizontally, the dependent half becomes bright red in contrast to the pale upper half. All three are benign.

Benign pustular dermatoses in neonates (1) *erythema toxicum neonatorum* - up to 70% of newborns, beginning on 2nd or 3rd day and lasting up to 2-3 weeks. 2-3 mm red blotchy macules and papules evolve to pustules with a red base. (2) *Transient neonatal pustular melanosis* - 4% of neonates, and is more common in black males. 2-5 mm pustules on a non-erythematous base are present at birth and found on the chin, neck, upper trunk, abdomen and thighs. (3) *Acropustulosis of infancy* - a chronic recurrent pustular eruption on palms and soles, with occasional involvement of the scalp, trunk, and extremities. Episodes last 1-3 weeks and can recur until age 3. During flare-ups, infants are fussy, and pruritis is severe. Sterile intradermal pustules occur. Topical steroids may relieve symptoms. (4) *Sebaceous gland hyperplasia* due to androgens is common on the nose and cheeks after birth. (5) *Miliaria* - obstruction of sweat flow with rupture of eccrine sweat glands due to heat with 1-2 mm vesicle crops on uninflamed skin at intertriginous areas: scalp, face, trunk. (6) *Milia* - pearly yellow 1-3 mm papules on face of 50% of newborns due to epidermal inclusion cysts from pilosebaceous cyst of vellus hair.

Scaling dermatitides include (1) *irritant contact dermatitis* - red, scaling rash involving the convex surfaces of perineum, lower abdomen, buttocks, and thighs with sparing of intertriginous areas. Secondary staphylococcal skin infection may occur. Treat with gentle cleaning, lubricants and barrier pastes (e.g., zinc oxide), and topical steroids. (2) *Candida* - bright red with sharp borders, satellite red papules and pustules, involvement of skin creases. Diagnose clinically or by KOH slide and treat with topical antifungals. (3) *seborrheic dermatitis* - salmon colored patches with greasy yellow scales beginning in intertriginous areas, diaper, axilla and scalp (cradle cap). May persist up to 8-12 months old. Treat with mild keratolytics (e.g. antiseborrheic shampoos, zinc pyrithione, sulfur and salicylic acid topical preparation. Emollients, topical antifungals, and low potency topical steroids may resolve skin lesions.

Select serious diseases causing rashes in newborn period include (1) *congenital syphilis* - skin lesions often begin between 2-6 weeks old with maculopapular eruption beginning on the palms and soles, later spreading to trunk. Smooth round, moist patches, involve the mouth and perianal area, while rhinitis with profuse and bloody rhinorrhea is often present. Systemic disease will manifest ....

as lymphadenopathy, pneumonitis, nephritis, enteritis, pancreatitis, meningitis, or osteochondritis. (2) *Acrodermatitis enteropathica* (AEP) - causes an erosive diaper dermatitis, diarrhea, and hair loss during the first few months of life. Weeping crusted red patches also appear with a perioral, acral and intertriginous distribution. Responds to oral or IV zinc. (3) Herpes simplex - incubation period is 2-21 days (mean 6 days). Rash consists of 1-2 mm clustered papules and vesicles, becoming pustular and denuded. First lesions develop on scalp after head delivery. Multiorgan involvement can occur. Diagnose via Tzanck smear.

Childhood Exanthems

An exanthem is an eruption of skin associated with systemic illness

Rubeola (measles) - Begins with a prodrome of upper respiratory symptoms including cough, conjunctivitis, and coryza (nasal congestion). Exanthem begins 14 days after exposure, starting behind the ears and the hairline and spreading from head to feet. It is red and maculopapular with discrete lesions that become confluent. Pneumonia is most common reason for admission. Modified measles may develop in partially immune host (e.g., if received IgG) causing prolonged prodrome, and less ill appearance. Live vaccine given within 72 hr or ISG within 6 days of exposure prevents disease. Patients are infectious until 4 after rash onset.

Rubella - Usually mild disease often causing subclinical illness. Main morbidity occurs through communicability (up to 7 days from onset of rash) to pregnant mother and fetus. URI prodrome with widespread lymphadenopathy, notably involving the postoccipital and postauricular nodes. Small macules coalesce on the trunk and fade by day three. Arthralgias are common.

Scarlet fever - Reaction to toxin produced by Group A streptococcal pharyngitis 12-48 hours after onset of sore throat. The rash is rough to touch, and appears first in skin folds (neck, groin, axilla, and antecubitum). Circumoral pallor occurs (sparing of area near mouth and nose). The rash blanches. 24 hours of antibiotics are necessary prior to becoming non-communicable.

Erythema infectiosum (fifth disease) - Parvovirus B19 is the etiology. The rash begins with bright red cheeks, then later a faint maculopapular pink rash on the trunk and extremities, clearing in lacy pattern. Transient anemia may occur.

Roseola (exanthem subitum) - Human herpes virus 6 is the etiology. Most common at ages 6 months to 3 years. The clinical course is characterized by sudden onset of a high fever, mild periorbital puffiness, conjunctivitis, and occasionally a febrile seizure. The rash begins as the fever declines. A faint pink, maculopapular (sometime pruritic) rash appears over trunk.

Papulosquamous Rashes

Disorder & Treatment	Skin lesions	Location
Atopic dermatitis *Emollients or Topical steroids*	Papules, vesicles, scales, lichenification	Flexure surfaces (extensor in infants), cheeks, forehead, face. Diaper area and creases are spared.
Contact dermatitis *Topical/Oral steroids*	Papules, vesicles, scales, and crusting	Face, trunk, extremities and especially exposed areas
Irritant dermatitis *Zinc oxide or Topical steroids*	Papules, vesicles, scales and crusting	face, trunk, extremities, especially convex surfaces, spares skin folds
Pityriasis rosea	Papules, scales	Christmas tree pattern on trunk
Psoriasis *Emollients, Topical steroids, UV light + Psoralen*	Round or oval red plaques with silvery scales	Scalp, trunk, extensor extremities, or areas of trauma. Nail pitting, dystrophy, and fissuring of palms and soles may be present.
Seborrheic dermatitis *Shampoo, Emollients, or Topical steroids*	Greasy scales, papules, erythema, pigment changes	Hair-bearing areas of face, scalp (cradle cap), axilla, inguinal areas, neck, and posterior auricular region
Syphilis *IV Antibiotics Penicillin*	Maculopapular, desquamation, vesicles, papules, warts, bullae	Maculopapular rash of palms/soles spreading to extremities & trunk; Moist warts (intertriginous, periorifice)
Tinea *Topical or Oral Antifungals*	Red scales, papules, pustules, vesicles	Non-hair-bearing areas of scalp, trunk and extremities

Treatment Options

Treatment	Options
Shampoo	antiseborrheic shampoos (e.g., *Head and Shoulders, Sebulex*)
Emollients	*Eucerin cream, Vaseline*
Oral antifungal	griseofulvin; see page 63
Oral steroids	prednisone, prednisolone; 1-2 mg/kg/day
Topical antifungals	clotrimazole, miconazole
Topical Steroids	hydrocortisone 0.5-1.0%, triamcinolone 0.1%

Vesiculopustular Rashes

Rash	Skin lesions	Location
Impetigo	Honey colored crusting or bullae	Face, trunk, extremities
Staphylococcal scalded skin syndrome (SSSS)	Generalized sunburn, circumoral erythema, periorifice crusting, Nikolsky's sign, sterile bullae	Total body with sparing of mucous membranes. Primary site of infection may be conjunctivae, nasopharynx, intertriginous area, umbilical stump, or circumcision.
Herpes simplex	Grouped thick-walled vesicles, pustules	Face, trunk, extremities, perineum, or mucous membranes
Herpes zoster	Grouped papules, vesicles, erosions	Dermatomal distribution
Erythema multiforme	Papules, wheals, target lesions	Generalized, palms, soles, with ≥ 2 mucous membranes involved in Stevens - Johnson syndrome
Toxic epidermal necrolysis	Generalized sunburn, sloughing, Nikolsky's sign	Generalized with mucous membrane involvement. Deeper epidermal cleavage plane than SSSS

Purpuric Rashes *(also see Bleeding Disorders, page 50)*

Rash	Skin lesions	Location
Idiopathic thrombocytopenic purpura	Petechiae, ecchymoses, hematomas	Exposed sites, bony prominences, and mucosa
Acute leukemia	Petechiae, purpura	Generalized, with adenopathy, hepatosplenomegaly, sternal tenderness
Aplastic anemia	Petechiae, purpura, ecchymoses with thick raised centers	Generalized or sites of injury
DIC	Petechiae, purpura, areas of skin necrosis	Generalized (petechiae tend to be palpable with *meningococcemia*)
Factor deficiency (e.g., hemophilia)	Ecchymoses with thick raised centers	Exposed areas or sites of injury (petechiae unusual)

Developmental Milestones

Age	Milestone
Newborn	• Lies flexed, turns head side to side, fixates to light and close objects
1 month	• More extended legs, responsive smile (6-8 weeks), follows object
4 months	• Lifts head/chest up, rolls front to back, reaches for objects, cooing
6 months	• Sits without support, pulls, bears some weight on legs, babbles
9 months	• Bears weight, stands holding on to furniture, crawls, says "mama/dada"
1 year	• Walks holding hand, pincer response, 3 words other than "mama"
2 years	• Climbs stairs, runs and jumps, uses spoon well, 3 word sentences
3 years	• Rides tricycle, briefly stands on foot, counts to 3, knows entire name
6 years	• Balances on foot, hops, counts to 10, 10 syllable sentences

Weight, Height, Head Circumference 5th, 50th, and 95th Percentiles

	Males				Females		
Age[1]	Height[2]	Weight[3]	HC[4]	Age[1]	Height[2]	Weight[3]	HC[4]
1 mo	50–55-59	3.2-4.3-5.4	35-37-40	1 mo	49-54-57	3.0-4.0-4.9	34-36-38
3 mo	57-61-65	4.4-6.0-7.4	38-41-43	3 mo	55-60-63	4.2-5.4-6.7	37-40-42
6 mo	63-68-72	6.2-7.9-9.5	42-44-46	6 mo	62-66-70	5.8-7.2-8.7	40-42-45
9 mo	68-72-77	7.5-9.2-10.9	44-46-48	9 mo	66-70-75	7-8.6-10.2	42-44-46
1 y	72-76-81	8.4-10.1-12	45-47-49	1 y	70-74-79	7.8-9.5-11	44-46-48
1.5 y	78-82-88	9.6-11.5-13.4	46-48-51	1.5 y	76-81-86	8.9-10.8-12.8	45-47-49
2 y	82-88-94	10.5-12.6-14.7	47-49-51	2 y	81-87-92	9.9-11.9-14.1	46-48-50
3 y	91-97-103	12.3-14.7-17.3	49-51-53	3 y	90-96-102	11.6-14-16.5	48-49-51
4 y	96-103-110	13.6-16.7-20.2	-	4 y	95-102-108	13.1-16-19.9	-
5 y	102-110-117	15.3-18.7-23.1	-	5 y	101-108-116	14.5-18-22.6	-

[1] y-years or mo-months, [2]Height-(cm), [3]Weight-kilograms, [4]HC- head circumference (cm)

United States Vital Statistics 1977 (Nov 165):I-IV; 1979: 1.

Other Growth Milestones

- **Dentition** – 1st teeth to erupt - lower incisors at 6 mo, central incisors (6-8 mo), lateral incisors (7-9 mo), 1st molar (12-14 mo), cuspids (16-18 mo), 2nd molars (20-24 mo). All 20 primary teeth erupt by 2 yr. Permanent teeth begin to erupt at 5-6 years, with all 32 erupting by teens.
- **Fontanelle** - Posterior fontanelle closes by 4 mo. Anterior fontanelle ↓ in size at 6 mo, closes at 9-18 mo. (Testing required if ant. fontanelle open after 18 mo)
- **Sinuses** - The ethmoid and maxillary sinuses are aerated at birth, while the frontal and sphenoid sinuses become aerated by 5-6 years.
- **Menarche** - Mean age of menarche is 12.7 years (11-16 range).
  1. Precocious puberty - onset of menses before age 10
  2. Primary amenorrhea – absence of menses beyond 16 years (always abnormal and requires evaluation)

Adrenal Disorders

Adrenal Insufficiency
Fever, vomiting, altered mental status, ↓BP, shock, ↓Na+, ↑K+, ↓glucose. Associated with chronic steroid use or unidentified adrenal disease (e.g., Addison's, congenital enzyme defects).

Adrenal Crisis Therapy
- If possible, draw and store blood sample for later steroid-level analyses
- 20 ml/kg normal saline bolus IV to correct shock (may repeat as needed)
- $D_{25}W$ (dextrose 25% in water), 2 ml/kg IV and Hydrocortisone 1-2 mg/kg IV
- Antibiotics if suspicion of sepsis (e.g., ceftriaxone 50 mg/kg)
- DOCA (deoxycorticosterone acetate) 1-2 mg IM (less urgent than other treatments)

Diabetes Mellitus

Diabetic ketoacidosis (DKA)

DKA causes 70% of diabetic related deaths under the age of 10 years. DKA is the 1st presentation of diabetes in 15-30%.

Typical Deficits in DKA		
	Fluid	• 10% body weight (BW)
	Na+	• 8-10 mEq/kg of BW
	Cl-	• 5-7 mEq/kg of BW
	K+	• 5 mEq/kg of BW

Treatment of DKA
- Apply cardiac monitor and administer O_2 if altered mental status or shock.
- Replace fluid and electrolyte deficits gradually over the first 24-48 hours.
- **The 1st hour:** Normal saline 10-20 ml/kg IV bolus (repeat prn to correct shock) Load insulin 0.1 units/kg IV.
- **1-9 hours:** After correcting hypotension, administer 50% of fluid deficit with 0.45% NS over next 8 hours. Consider 0.9% NS if 1st serum Na+ < 135 mEq/L.
- **10-24 hours:** Replace the remaining 50% fluid deficit over this time period.
- **Add dextrose** to the IV fluids when the glucose falls to < 250-300 mg/dl.
- **Replace K+** (if OK urine output) and phosphate. Phosphate shifts O_2 dissociation curve to the right (increasing O_2 delivery to tissues and correcting acidosis). Replace K+ with approximately 50/50 mix of KCL and K_3PO_4.

If serum potassium is	Potassium in IV fluids
<3 mEq/l	40-60 mEq/l
3-4 mEq/l	30 mEq/l
4-5 mEq/l	20 mEq/l
5-6 mEq/l	≤ 10 mEq/l

- **Insulin:** Infusion of approximately 0.1 units/kg/hour. Change to subcutaneous insulin when pH >7.30 and monitor hourly glucose. If glucose drops to 250 mg/dl, reduce the rate of insulin administration to 0.02-0.05 units/kg/hour.

Criteria for outpatient treatment of DKA

- Initial glucose <500 and *either* a pH ≥ 7.2 or a bicarbonate ≥ 10 mEq/L (have > 90% chance of resolving metabolic parameters within 3 hours.)
- pH ≥ 7.35 and bicarbonate ≥ 20 mEq/L after 3 hours of treatment
- Resolution of significant symptoms and vital sign abnormalities
- Reliable parents, older patient, and closely coordinated follow-up

Bonadio: Am J Dis Child 1988; 142:448

Other Complications of Diabetes and Therapy

- *Cerebral edema* is unpredictable in onset with ↓ mental status, coma, and pupillary changes 8-12 hours after initiation of DKA therapy. Mortality is > 90%. Treat with mannitol, intubation, and hyperventilation. Rapid fluid administration and total fluids >4 l/m²/day are associated with development of this disorder.
- *Hyperosmolar coma* is very rare in children and is associated with preexisting neurologic disorders. Fluids and management of underlying cause are primary treatment modalities. Only 10-50% of the insulin dose used in DKA is needed.

Hypoglycemia

Hypoglycemia

Hypoglycemia is defined as a blood glucose < 40-45 mg/dl (< 30 mg/dl in neonate). Hypoglycemia is ketotic in > 50% case. It is most commonly due to poor nutrition or overmedication with insulin or hypoglycemic agents.

Etiology of Hypoglycemia

• ↓ Intake (vomiting, malnutrition)	• Excess endogenous insulin (e.g., islet cell tumors)
• ↓Absorption (diarrhea,malabsorption)	
• Inborn errors of metabolism (amino acid, glycogen storage, or glucose metabolic enzyme deficiencies)	• Insulin or oral hypoglycemic excess
	• *Endocrine disorder*: Hypopituitarism, hypothyroidism, adrenal insufficiency
• Sepsis, Reye's syndrome	• Poison (aspirin, β-blockers, alcohol)

Evaluation

History: Fed hypoglycemia (< 4-6 h after meal) is associated with GI tract disease (poor absorption), and early diabetes while *fasting* hypoglycemia (> 5-6 h after meal) is associated with insulin secreting tumors, and endocrine disorders.

Dipstick urine for ketones. Absence of ketones suggests hyperinsulinemia (medication or tumor) or defect in fatty acid oxidation.

Management of Hypoglycemia

Age	Dose and Concentration	Other Treatment
0-30 days	• 10 ml/kg of D₁₀W IV	• glucagon 0.1-0.2 mg/kg IM
1-24 months	• 4 ml/kg of D₂₅W IV	• diazoxide IV if severe
> 2 years	• 2 ml/kg of D₅₀W IV	persistent hypoglycemia

Environmental Disorders

Minor Heat Illness

- *Heat Syncope*: Postural hypotension from vasodilation, volume depletion, and ↓ vascular tone. Rehydrate, remove from heat, and evaluate for serious disease.
- *Heat cramps*: Painful, contractions of calves, thigh, or shoulders in those who are sweating liberally and drinking hypotonic solutions (e.g. water). Replace fluids: 0.1-0.2% NS oral solution or IV NS rehydration. Do not use salt tablets.
- *Heat Exhaustion*: Salt and water depletion causing orthostasis, and hyperthermia (usually < 104F). Mental status, and neurologic exam are normal. Lab: high hematocrit, high sodium, or high BUN. Treat with NS 10-20 ml/kg IV.

Heatstroke

Clinical Features	Risk Factors
<ul><li>Hyperpyrexia (temp. > 104-105.8F)</li><li>Central nervous system dysfunction (seizures, altered mentation, plantar responses, hemiplegia, ataxia)</li><li>Loss of sweating (variably present)</li></ul>	<ul><li>Very young or old age</li><li>Drugs that limit sweating (anticholinergics, amphetamines, cocaine, antihypertensive agents)</li></ul>

Complications of heatstroke: rhabdomyolysis, renal or liver failure, ↓ Na, ↓ Ca, ↓ phosphate, ↓ or ↑ K and disseminated intravascular coagulation.

Management of Heatstroke

- Administer oxygen, protect airway if comatose or seizing. Check blood glucose.
- Measure temperature with continuous rectal probe accurate at high levels.
- Begin IV NS cautiously as pulmonary edema is common and mean fluid requirement is < 20 ml/kg in 1st 4 hours. Consider central line pressures as guide.
- Immediate cooling by: (1) *evaporation*: Spray with tepid water and direct fan at patient (0.1 - 0.3C/min temp. drop). For shivering, IV lorazepam 0.05-0.1 mg/kg IV or (2) *ice water (or 60F) tub immersion*: (*controversial*) (temp. drop ~ 0.16C/min). (3) *Ice packs, cooling blankets, peritoneal dialysis, gastric lavage* with cold water are slow or unproven. (4) Avoid aspirin (hyperpyrexia). Avoid repeated Tylenol doses (possible liver damage and ineffective in heatstroke)
- Stop above measures at temperature of 102-104 to avoid over-correction.
- Place Foley catheter to monitor urine output (see rhabdomyolysis page 29).
- Obtain CBC, electrolytes, renal function, glucose, liver enzymes, LDH/CPK, PT, and PTT, arterial blood gas, and fibrin degradation products. ECG and CXR.
- Exclude other fever cause: infection, malignant hyperthermia, thyroid, drugs, etc

Other Heat Related Disorders

- **Malignant hyperthermia (MH)**: Autosomal dominant. Fever, + muscle rigidity after anesthetics or succinylcholine. *Treatment*: Stop agent, lower temperature as in heatstroke (avoid phenothiazines), give dantrolene 2-3 mg/kg IV (max 10 mg/kg).

- **Neuroleptic Malignant Syndrome:** Similar to MH with fever, muscle rigidity, and altered mentation, but due to anticholinergics (e.g. phenothiazines). *Treatment:* Stop agent, treat heatstroke (avoid phenothiazines) and administer dantrolene 2-3 mg/kg IV (max 10 mg/kg) and bromocriptine 2.5-10 mg PO tid.

- **Rhabdomyolysis:** Syndrome with release of contents into circulation due to tissue hypoxia, direct injury, exercise, enzyme defects, metabolic disease (DKA, ↓ K, ↓ Na, or ↓ phosphate, thyroid), toxins, infections, heatstroke. *Complications:* renal failure,↑K,↑Ca or↓ Ca,↑or↓phosphate,↑ uric acid, compartment syndrome, DIC. *Treatment*: (1) IV NS to keep UO[1] > 2-3 ml/kg/hr, (2) Alkalinize urine, (3) Mannitol if poor UO: 0.25-0.5 g/kg IV, + add 12.5 g to each L NS, (4) Dialyze ↑K+, or uremia.

UO[1] – urine output

HYPOTHERMIA

Severity	Temp. F (C)	Features
Mild	91-95 (33-35)	Maximal shivering + slurred speech at < 95°F
Moderate	85-90 (29-32)	At < 89°F altered mental status, mydriasis, shivering ceases, muscles are rigid, incoordination, bradypnea
Severe	≤ 82 (≤ 28)	Bradycardia in 50%, Osborne waves on EKG, voluntary motion stops, pupils are fixed and dilated
	79 (26)	Loss of consciousness, areflexia, no pain response
	77 (25)	No respirations, appear dead, pulmonary edema
	68 (20)	Asystole

Management of Hypothermia

- No vigorous manipulation or active external rewarming unless mild hypothermia
- Evaluate for cause (e.g. sepsis, hypoglycemia, CNS disease, adrenal crisis).
- **Mild hypothermia** (> 32°C): Administer humidified warmed O_2. Passive external rewarming and treatment of underlying disease is often only treatment needed.
- **Moderate hypothermia** (29-32°C): Active internal rewarming. Drugs & cardioversion for cardiac arrest may be ineffective. Warm humidified O_2, with gastric or peritoneal lavage if < 1C/hour temperature rise. Perform CPR, and advanced life support prn.
- **Severe hypothermia** (≤ 29°C): (1) Warm humidified O_2, and warm IV fluids. (2) If nonarrested, warmed peritoneal dialysis (41C dialysate), or (3) pleural irrigation (41C). (4) If core temperature < 25C consider fermoral-femoral bypass. (5) Use open pleural lavage for direct cardiac rewarming if core temperature < 28C after 1 h of bypass in an arrest rhythm. (6) If signs of life, and non-arrested, avoid CPR, and ACLS. If cardiac arrest, CPR and ACLS are OK. (6) Use bretylium 5mg/kg for ventricular fib. Do not treat atrial arrhythmies. (7) Use NS to treat hypotension. Use pressors cautiously prn. (8) Consider empiric D_{50}, Narcan 2mg IV, + hydrocortisone 100 mg IV in all.

Snake Bite Envenomation

Grade	Features	Antivenin dose
None	± Fang marks, no pain, erythema or systemic symptoms	None
Mild[1]	Fang marks, mild pain/edema, no systemic symptoms	0-5 vials (50 ml)
Moderate	Fang marks, severe pain, moderate edema in 1st 12 h, mild symptoms (vomiting, paresthesias), mild coagulopathy (without bleeding)	10 vials (100 ml)
Severe	Fang marks, severe pain/edema, severe symptoms (hypotension, respiratory distress), coagulopathy with bleeding	15-20 vials (150-200 ml)

[1]Controversial – some experts recommend no antivenin for mild envenomation.

Prehospital Treatment for Crotalid Envenomation

- Decrease patient movement, and transport to nearest medical facility.
- Immobilize extremity in neutral position below level of heart.
- Incision + drainage and tourniquets are unproven and not recommended.

Emergency Treatment for Crotalid Envenomation

- Perform examination, measure site of envenomation so repeated assessments can be made. Resuscitate with fluids, pressors as needed.
- If significant envenomation, obtain baseline CBC, electrolytes, renal and liver function tests, PT, PTT, fibrinogen, urinalysis, ECG, and type and cross.
- If no signs of envenomation, cleanse wound, administer tetanus prophylaxis and observe for a minimum of 6 hours.
- Perform skin test only if antivenin to be administered: 0.2 ml SC (diluted 1:10 with NS) at a site distant from bite. Observe for signs of allergy for at least 10 minutes after injection. A negative reaction does not entirely exclude allergy.
- Need for antivenin and specific dose is controversial. Prior to administration, obtain consent, expand vascular volume with NS, premedicate with diphenhydramine 1 mg/kg IV, and dilute antivenin in 50-100 ml for each vial.

Antivenin Administration (see dose above)

- Start infusion at slow rate for 15 min. If no allergy, increase rate so that infusion takes 1-2 hours. If symptoms progress, additional antivenin may be required.
- If allergic reaction and antivenin is still necessary, start arterial line, continue to treat with NS ± albumin, administer methylprednisolone 2 mg/kg IV, and diphenhydramine 1 mg/kg IV. Hang epinephrine drip in line separate from antivenin (eg. 0.6 mg/kg epi 1:1,000 in 100 ml NS), and maximally dilute antivenin. Begin antivenin slowly. If needed begin epi drip at low dose [1 ml/hr of above mixture = 0.1 µg/kg/min] Once sympathetic response and allergic reaction gone, restart antivenin slowly. If allergy contact local poison center.

Elapidae (Coral Snake) Envenomation

This species is found in the southeast US and Arizona.These, snakes must bite and chew. Local effects + bite marks may be minimal. Symptoms are primarily systemic: altered mentation, cranial nerve deficits, muscle weakness, and respiratory failure. Symptoms may be delayed up to 24 h. Admit all for possible respiratory or neurologic deterioration. All require Coral Snake Antivenin. *Dose of antivenin*: 3-6 vials administered as crotalidae antivenin. Sonoran (Arizona) coral snake venom is less toxic, no deaths have been reported, and coral snake antivenin is ineffective.

Special Situations

Mojave rattlesnake: May cause muscle weakness, paralysis, or respiratory failure with few local symptoms. Empiric crotalid antivenin is indicated in most instances.
Exotic snakes: Call **(602) 626-6016** for information regarding available anti-venin.
Serum sickness will develop in most receiving > 5 vials of antivenin within 5-20 days causing joint pain, myalgias, and possibly rash. Warn patient and treat with diphenhydramine (*Benadryl*) 1 mg/kg PO q4-6 h and prednisone 1-2 mg/kg PO qd.

Spider Bites

Black Widow - Found throughout US, but more common in South. Females have 1.5cm length (5 cm with legs), males are 1/3 size (and non-toxic). Only 1 of 5 species has orange red hour-glass on its abdomen. *Clinical features*: Mild to moderately painful bite. In 1 h, redness, swelling, and cramps begin at the bite and gradually spread. Abdominal wall involvement can mimic peritonitis. 10-30% are hypertensive, and rare cases of shock, coma and respiratory failure occur.
Treatment: (1) O_2, IV access, & cardiac monitoring. (2) Calcium gluconate 10%, 1 ml/kg (max 10 ml) slow IV. (2) Lorazepam (*Ativan*) 0.05-0.1 mg/kg IV .

Indications for Admission and Antivenin Administration (controversial)

Respiratory or cardiac symptoms	Protracted distress despite calcium, lorazepam
Pregnancy with symptoms	Symptomatic and < 12 years
History hypertension, cardiovas-	Marked hypertension
cular disease.	*Emerg Med Clin North Am* 1992; 269

(3) Administer 1-2 vials of antivenin IV diluted in 50-100 ml NS. Skin testing is recommended, allergy can occur, and serum sickness may follow administration.
Brown Recluse: Found mostly in southern US, and in dark places (attics, wood piles etc.). Bites are mild and cause ulcerative necrosis hours to days later. Lesions are red, and blanch, later evolving to blue-gray macule with central ulcer. Blisters may form. Systemic symptoms: arthralgias, GI upset, hemoglobinuria (renal failure), DIC, and shock. *Treatment*: (1) Wound care, tetanus, antibiotics if infection. (2) Excise wound if > 2 cm, and well established borders (usually 2-3 wk after bite). (3) Dapsone is not recommended in children. (4) Hyperbaric O_2 may be useful.

Electrolyte Disorders

Formulas

Anion Gap	• Na^+ - (Cl^- + HCO_3^-) *Normal* = 8-16 mEq/L
Osmolal gap	• measured – calculated osmolality *Normal* = 0-10 mOsm/L
Calculated Osmolality	• $2xNa^+$ +(glucose/18) + (BUN/2.8) + (ethanol/4.6)+ (methanol/2.6) + (ethylene glycol/5) + (acetone/5.5) + (isopropanol/5.9)

Causes of ↑Anion Gap	*Causes of ↓Anion Gap*	*Causes of ↑Osmol Gap*
Methanol	Lactate	Alcohols (methanol,
Uremia	Ethanol,ethylene	ethylene glycol,
Diabetes	glycol	isopropanol)
Paraldehyde	Salicylates,	Sugars (glycerol,
Iron, INH	starvation	mannitol)
		Ketones (acetone)

	Primary Disorder	*Normal Compensation*
Acid Base Rules of Compensation	Metabolic Acidosis	PCO_2 = (1.5 x HCO_3^- + 8) ± 2
	Acute Respiratory Acidosis	↑ΔHCO_3^- = (0.1 x ΔPCO_2↑)
	Chronic Respiratory Acidosis	↑ΔHCO_3^- = (0.4 x ΔPCO_2↑)
	Metabolic Alkalosis	PCO_2 = (0.9 x HCO_3^- + 9) ± 2
	Acute Respiratory Alkalosis	↓ΔHCO_3^- = (0.2 x ΔPCO_2↓)
	Chronic Respiratory Alkalosis	↓ΔHCO_3^- = (0.4 x ΔPCO_2↓)

High Yield Criteria for Electrolyte Ordering in the ED	• Age ≤ 6 months	• Diabetes mellitus
	• Vomiting	• Dry mucous membranes
	• Tachycardia	• Capillary refill > 2 seconds

Presence of any criteria was 100% sensitive in detecting significant abnormalities.
Acad Emerg Med 1997; 4:1025.

CALCIUM

Hypocalcemia - Total calcium < 8.5 mg/dl   or ionized Ca^{+2} < 2.0 mEq/L (1.0 mmol/L)
Hypercalcemia - Total calcium > 10.5 mg/dl or ionized Ca^{+2} > 2.7 mEq/L (1.3 mmol/L)

Hypoalbuminemia correction	• Subtract 0.8 mg/dl from total serum Ca^{+2} for each 1 g/dl ↓ in serum albumin below normal

Hypocalcemia – Clinical Features

Symptoms	Physical Findings	Electrocardiogram
Paresthesias, fatigue	Hyperactive reflexes	• Prolonged QT
Seizures, tetany	Chvostek(C)/Trousseau(T) signs[1]	(esp. Ca^{+2} < 6.0 mg/dl)
Vomiting, weakness	Low blood pressure	• Bradycardia,
Laryngospasm	Congestive heart failure	• Arrhythmias

[1]C–muscle twitch with tap facial nerve, T–carpal spasm after forearm BP cuff up for 3 min

Hypocalcemia Etiology [1,2]

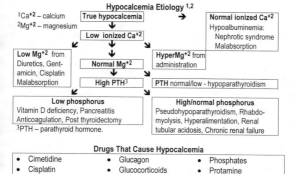

[1]Ca^{+2} – calcium
[2]Mg^{+2} – magnesium

True hypocalcemia	→	Normal ionized Ca^{+2}

Normal ionized Ca^{+2}
Hypoalbuminemia:
  Nephrotic syndrome
  Malabsorption

Low ionized Ca^{+2}

Low Mg^{+2} from
Diuretics, Gent-
amicin, Cisplatin
Malabsorption

Normal Mg^{+2}

HyperMg^{+2} from
administration

High PTH[3]

PTH normal/low - hypoparathyroidism

Low phosphorus
Vitamin D deficiency, Pancreatitis
Anticoagulation, Post thyroidectomy
[3]PTH – parathyroid hormone.

High/normal phosphorus
Pseudohypoparathyroidism, Rhabdomyolysis, Hyperalimentation, Renal
tubular acidosis, Chronic renal failure

Drugs That Cause Hypocalcemia

- Cimetidine
- Cisplatin
- Citrate (transfusion)
- Dilantin, phenobarbital
- Gentamicin, Tobramycin

- Glucagon
- Glucocorticoids
- Heparin
- Loop diuretics (*Lasix*)
- Magnesium sulfate

- Phosphates
- Protamine
- Norepinephrine
- Sodium nitroprusside
- Theophylline

Hypocalcemia Treatment

Check serum electrolytes, BUN, creatinine, albumin, magnesium, arterial pH

Drug	Preparation	Route	Drug Dose (max. dose)[3]
Ca gluconate	10% solution –100mg/ml	IM, IV[1,2]	0.5-1 ml/kg (5-10 ml)
Ca chloride	10% solution –100mg/ml	IV[1,2]	0.2-0.3 ml/kg (5-10 ml)
Ca gluconate	500, 650, 975, 1000mg (10%)	PO	100 mg/kg qid (500 mg/kg)
Ca glubionate	0.5-1 g tab, 1.8 g/5 ml	PO	0.6-2 g/kg/d divided qid (9g/d)

[1] Administer IV calcium (Ca) slowly (over ≥ 5-10 min) while patient on cardiac monitor. IV calcium may cause hypotension, tissue necrosis, bradycardia or digoxin toxicity.

[2] Consider central administration to prevent tissue damage. Local infiltration of hyaluronidase reverses necrosis.

[3] All doses are doses of drug and not of calcium.

Hypercalcemia – Clinical Features

General	• Weakness, polydipsia, dehydration
Neurologic	• Confusion, irritability, hyporeflexia, headache
Skeletal	• Bone pain, fractures
Cardiac	• Hypertension, QT shortening, wide T wave, arrhythmia
GI	• Anorexia, weight loss, constipation, ulcer, pancreatitis
Urologic	• Polyuria, renal insufficiency, nephrolithiasis

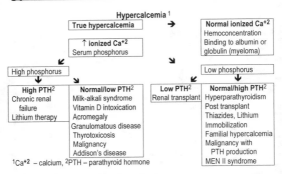

Hypercalcemia [1]

True hypercalcemia	→	Normal ionized Ca[+2]

↑ ionized Ca[+2]
Serum phosphorus

Normal ionized Ca[+2]
Hemoconcentration
Binding to albumin or globulin (myeloma)

| High phosphorus | | | Low phosphorus |

High PTH[2]	Normal/low PTH[2]	Low PTH[2]	Normal/high PTH[2]
Chronic renal failure Lithium therapy	Milk-alkali syndrome Vitamin D intoxication Acromegaly Granulomatous disease Thyrotoxicosis Malignancy Addison's disease	Renal transplant	Hyperparathyroidism Post transplant Thiazides, Lithium Immobilization Familial hypercalcemia Malignancy with PTH production MEN II syndrome

[1]Ca[+2] – calcium, [2]PTH – parathyroid hormone

Hypercalcemia Management

- Especially important for Ca[+2] > 12 mg/dl, hypotension, or cardiac arrhythmias
- IV NS 20 ml/kg with repeat boluses to keep urine output > 2-3 ml/kg/hour
- Furosemide 1-2 mg/kg to promote caluresis (after adequate hydration)
- Consider IV hydrocortisone (1-2 mg/kg) if sarcoid, vitamin A or D toxicity, or leukemia, mithramycin (metastatic bone disease), calcitonin and dialysis may also be useful

MAGNESIUM

Hypomagnesemia (<1.5 mEq/L) Due to diuretics, aminoglycosides, cyclosporine. Irritable muscle, tetany, seizure, arrhythmia. Treat: $MgSO_4$ 5-10 mg/kg IV over 20 min.
Hypermagnesemia (>2.2 mEq/L) Due to renal failure, excess maternal Mg supplement, or overuse of Mg-containing medicine. Clinical features: weakness, hyporeflexia, paralysis, and EKG with AV block & QT prolongation. Treat: $CaCl$ (10%) 0.2-0.3 ml/kg (max 5 ml) IV.

POTASSIUM

Acute decreases in pH will increase K[+] (a ↓ pH of 0.1 will ↑K[+] 0.3-1.3 mEq/L).
Acute metabolic acid base disorders cause most changes.

Hypokalemia

Causes of Hypokalemia	
• *Decreased K[+] intake* • *Intracellular shift* (normal stores): alkalemia, insulin, pseudohypokalemia of leukemia, familial hypokalemic periodic paralysis (HPP).	• *Increased excretion*: diuretics, hyperaldosteronism, penicillins (exchange Na[+]/K[+]), sweating, diarrhea (colonic fluid has high K[+]), vomiting (compensation for metabolic alkalosis)

Clinical Features of Hypokalemia	Treatment of Hypokalemia
• Lethargy, confusion weakness • Areflexia, difficult respirations • Autonomic instability, Low BP	• Ensure good urine output first • If mild, replace orally only • Parenteral K+ if severe hypokalemia (e.g. cardiac or neuromuscular symptoms or DKA).
EKG findings in Hypokalemia	
• K+ ≤ 3.0 mEq/L: low voltage QRS, flat T waves, ↓ ST segment, prominent P and U waves • K+ ≤ 2.5 mEq/L: prominent U wave • K+ ≤ 2.0 mEq/L: widened QRS	• Administer K+ no faster than 0.5-1.0 mEq/kg/hour using ≤ 40 mEq/L (cautiously while on cardiac monitor)

Hyperkalemia
Causes of Hyperkalemia

• *Pseudohyperkalemia* due to blood samples or hemolysis • *Exogenous:* blood, salt substitutes, potassium containing drugs (e.g. penicillin derivatives), acute digoxin toxicity, β blockers, succinylcholine	• *Endogenous* – acidemia, trauma, burns, rhabdomyolysis, DIC, sickle cell crisis, GI bleed, chemotherapy (destroying tumor mass), mineralocorticoid deficiency, congenital defects (21 hydroxylase deficiency)

Clinical Features of Hyperkalemia	Treatment of Hyperkalemia
• Paresthesias, weakness • Ascending paralysis sparing head, trunk, and respiration	• Calcium chloride (10%) to stabilize membrane – 0.1-0.3 ml/kg (max 5 ml) IV over 2-5 min, ± repeat q 5 min x 2
EKG in Hyperkalemia (K+ in mEq/L)	• NaHCO3 1-2 mEq/kg IV, may repeat
• K+ 5-6.0: peak T waves • K+ 6-6.5:↑ PR and QT intervals • K+ 6.5-7:↓ P, ↓ ST segments • K+ 7-7.5:↑ intraventricular conduction • K+ 7.5-8:↑ QRS widens, ST and T waves merge • K+ > 10: sine wave appearance	• Glucose 0.5-1.0 g/kg IV + insulin 1 unit/3g glucose IV (transcellular shift) • Albuterol nebulizer 1 cc, may repeat • Furosemide 1 mg/kg IV • Kayexalate 1 g/kg orally or rectally (lowers K+ 1.2 mEq/L in 4-6 hours) • Dialysis

SODIUM

Daily Na+ requirements: 1-2 mEq/kg/d in newborn and 3-4 mEq/kg/d - premature.

FE$_{Na}$ = fraction of Na+ in urine filtered by the glomerulus and not reabsorbed.

FE$_{Na}$ = 100 x (urine Na+/plasma Na+) / (urine creatinine/plasma creatinine)

Normal FE$_{Na}$ is < 3%, except under 2 months of age when FE$_{Na}$ up may be to 5%.

Hyponatremia

Pseudohyponatremia occurs with ↑glucose, ↑triglyceride and ↑protein.
Na^+ = falsely ↓ 1.6 mEq/L for each 100 mg/dL ↑ in glucose over 100 mg/dL.

Clinical Features of Hyponatremia	
• Lethargy, apathy	• Cerebral edema
• Depressed reflexes, muscle cramps	• Seizures
• Pseudobulbar palsies	• Hypothermia

Hyponatremia Etiology, Diagnosis, Management

Deficit body Na^+ > deficit body water		Excess total body water (no edema)		Excess total body water > excess Na^+ (edema)
Renal losses: diuretics, mineralocorticoid deficiency, salt losing nephritis, bicarbonaturia, ketonuria, osmotic diuresis	*Extrarenal loss:* vomit, diarrhea, 3rd space fluids, pancreatitis, peritonitis, traumatized muscle	Glucocorticoid deficiency, low thyroid, pain, emotional stress, drugs, (SIADH - U_{osm} usually > S_{osm})	Nephrotic syndrome, cirrhosis, CHF	Acute and chronic renal failure
↓	↓	↓	↓	↓
(Diagnosis – Urine labs)				
Na^+>20 mEq/L ↑FE$_{Na}$, ↓ SG[1] U_{osm}[3] varies	Na^+<10 mEq/L ↓FE$_{Na}$, ↑ SG[1] U_{osm}[3] > 800	Na^+>20 mEq/L NI[2] FE$_{Na}$, ↑ SG[1] U_{osm}[3] varies	Na^+<10 mEq/L ↓FE$_{Na}$, ↑ SG[1] high U_{osm}[3]	Na^+>20 mEq/L ↑FE$_{Na}$, ↓ SG[1] U_{osm}[3] varies
↓	↓	↓	↓	↓
Management				
Isotonic saline	Isotonic saline	Water restrict	Water restrict	Water restrict

[1] SG – specific gravity, [2] NI- normal, [3] U_{osm} – urine osmalality, [4] S_{osm} -serum osmolality

Hypertonic Saline Administration
• Only use in severe ↓ Na^+(<120 mEq/L) with seizures, or other life threats
• Administer 4 ml/kg 3% saline, at ≤ 1-2 ml/kg/hour OR bolus over 20 minutes
• 1 ml/kg of 3% saline raises serum Na by 1 mEq/L

Hypernatremia

Clinical Features of Hypernatremia	
• Lethargy, irritability, coma	• Doughy skin
• Seizures	• Late preservation of intravascular volume (and vital signs)
• Spasticity, hyperreflexia	

Hypernatremia Etiology, Diagnosis, Management

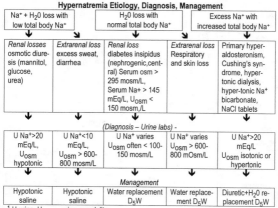

$Na^+ + H_2O$ loss with low total body Na^+		H_2O loss with normal total body Na^+		Excess Na^+ with increased total body Na^+
Renal losses osmotic diuresis (mannitol, glucose, urea)	*Extrarenal loss* excess sweat, diarrhea	*Renal loss* diabetes insipidus (nephrogenic,central) Serum osm > 295 mosm/L, Serum Na^+ > 145 mEq/L, U_{osm} < 150 mosm,/L	*Extrarenal loss* Respiratory and skin loss	Primary hyper-aldosteronism, Cushing's syndrome, hyper-tonic dialysis, hyper-tonic Na^+ bicarbonate, NaCl tablets

(Diagnosis – Urine labs) -

U Na^+>20 mEq/L, U_{osm} hypotonic	U Na^+<10 mEq/L, U_{osm} > 600-800 mosm/L	U Na^+ varies U_{osm} often < 100-150 mosm/L	U Na^+ varies U_{osm} > 600-800 mOsm/L	U Na^+>20 mEq/L U_{osm} isotonic or hypertonic

Management

Hypotonic saline	Hypotonic saline	Water replacement D_5W	Water replacement D_5W	Diuretic+H_2O replacement D_5W

[1] U-urine, U_{osm} – urine osmolality

Management of Hypernatremia

- Correct hypernatremia slowly over approximately 48 hours. Overvigorous rehydration causes cerebral edema, seizures, coma, or death. Lower Na^+ no faster than 1-2 mEq/L/hour.
- With endogenous Na^+ overload, treatment consists of salt restriction and correction of the primary underlying disorder. If there is excess exogenous mineralocorticoid, restrict salt and modify replacement therapy.
- Desmopressin (DDAVP) is indicated in children with diabetes insipidus. Intranasal DDAVP dose - 1.25-10 µg q day or bid.

Fluid Homeostasis

Pediatric IV maintenance fluids by weight:
   4 ml/kg/h **or** 100 ml/kg/day for first 10 kg, plus
   2 ml/kg/h **or** 50 ml/kg/day for second 10 kg, plus
   1 ml/kg/h **or** 20 ml/kg/day for all further kg
Maintenance fluids by BSA (body surface area) = 2,000 ml/m^2/day.
Normal BSA = square root of [height(cm) x weight (kg) / 3600]
Na^+ requirements = 3 mEq per liter of extracellular fluid per day, with liters of
   extracellular fluid calculated by multiplying weight in kg times 0.6.
K^+ requirements = 2 mEq per liter of intracellular fluid per day, with liters of
   intracellular fluid calculated by multiplying weight in kg times 0.4.

Clinical Findings in Dehydration

Findings	Mild(<5%)	Moderate (5-10%)	Severe (>10%)
appearance	alert	restless	limp, cold, acrocyanosis
heart rate	normal	rapid weak	thready
respirations	normal	deep, increased	deep and rapid
blood pressure	normal	normal or low	low
skin turgor	normal	slow retraction	retraction > 2 sec
eyes	normal	sunken	grossly sunken
tears	present	absent	absent
mucous membranes	moist	dry	very dry
urine output	normal	reduced, dark	minimal
urine specific gravity	≤ 1.020	~ 1.030	> 1.035
BUN	normal	elevated	very high
arterial pH	> 7.30	7.00 - 7.30	< 7.10
fluid deficit	40-50 ml/kg	60-90 ml/kg	100 ml/kg or more

Detection of dehydration	**High Yield Criteria for > 5% dehydration**
The presence of ≥ 2 of 4 high-yield criteria is 87% sensitive in detecting > 5% dehydration. *Acad Emerg Med 1996;395*	• Capillary refill > 2 seconds • Dry mucous membranes • Absent tears • General ill appearance

Dehydration – Clinical Features and Management

Classification	Isotonic	Hypotonic	Hypertonic
Sodium (mEq/L)	130-150	< 130	> 150
Cause	Usually GI[1] and ECF[2] fluid loss	Dilute fluid (water) replacement	Incorrectly diluted formula or high Na[+2] intake. ICF[3] loss exceeds ECF.
Deficit	Na[+2] = water loss	Na[+2] > water loss	Water > Na[+2] loss
Examination			
Blood pressure	Depressed	Very depressed	May be preserved
Heart rate	Increased	Increased	Minimal increase
Skin turgor	Poor	Very poor	Fair
Skin consistency	Dry	Clammy	Doughy
Mental status	Lethargy	Coma or seizure	Irritable or seizure
Initially Rehydrate with following[4]	Normal saline	Normal saline	D_5 ½NS with K+
Unique feature	The most common type of dehydration

Oral rehydration is appropriate for children with < 5 to 10% dehydration if they are able to take liquids by mouth | Consider 3% NS if severe or life-threatening symptoms (see page 36 for indications and dosing) | NS use can para-doxically ↑ Na+ Lower Na+ at < 2 mEq/L/h or < 10 mEq/L/24 h. Too rapid correction can cause CNS edema, CHF and renal damage. May be accompan-ied by ↓ Ca[+2] |
| Remember to exclude hypoglycemia in all cases | | | Assume 4ml/kg free water deficit for every 1 mEq/L Na+ > 145 |

[1] GI – gastrointestinal, [2] ECF – extracellular fluid, [3] ICF – intracellular fluid

[4] Use NS to reverse shock in all cases

Composition of Oral and Intravenous Solutions

Solution	Sodium (mEq/l)	Potassium (mEq/l)	Chloride (mEq/l)	Bicarbonate (mEq/l)[1]	Glucose (g/dl)
Extracellular fluid	142	4	103	27	~0.1
0.9NS	154	0	154	0	0
D5NS	154	0	154	0	5
Hypertonic 3%NS	513	0	513	0	0
0.45 NS	77	0	77	0	0
0.3NS	51	0	51	0	0
0.2NS	34	0	34	0	0
LR	130	0	109	28	0
D5LR	130	0	109	28	5
Infant Carvajal's[2]	81	0	61	20	4.65
Child Carvajal's[2]	132	3.8	109	27	4.8
WHO solution[3]	90	20	80	na	2.0
Lytren	50	25	45	30	2.0
Pedialyte	45	20	35	30	2.5
Rehydralyte	75	20	65	30	2.5
Resol	50	20	50	34	2.0
Ricelyte	50	25	45	10	3.0
Infalyte	50	20	40	na	2.0
Gatorade	28	2	na	na	2.1
Ginger ale	4	0.2	na	na	9.0
Coke	3	0.1	13.4	10.0	10.5
Pepsi	2	0.9	7.3	10.0	10.5
Apple juice	1-4	15-20	-	-	12.0
Grape juice	2-4	20-30	-	-	15.0
Jello	24	1.5	-	-	15.8

1 Or citrate or lactate. [2]Used for burns and contains 12.5 g/L albumin.
3 Excess amounts of the WHO (World Health Organization) formula have caused hypernatremia, therefore give this solution with free water.

Oral Rehydration Therapy	**WHO Recommendations**
Wheat and rice-based oral electrolyte solutions are superior to glucose solutions for rehydration, decrease stool frequency and volume.	• 1st hydrate with 100 ml/kg WHO formula over 4 h • Then 50 ml/kg of water or breast milk over next 2h • If still dehydrated, 50 ml/kg of WHO formula next 6h • Then 100 ml/kg of WHO formula over next 24 h, followed by 150 ml/kg/day of WHO formula • Give additional free H_2O with WHO formula or hypernatremia may occur

Gastrointestinal Disorders

Common GI Therapeutic Agents

Drug	Available forms	Dosing
bisacodyl (*Dulcolax, fleet enema*)	Enema: 10mg/30ml Supp: 5,10 mg Tab: 5 mg	Oral: 5 mg/dose Rectal (≤ 2 years): 5 mg/dose Rectal (> 2 years): 10 mg/dose
cimetidine (*Tagamet*)	Injectable: 150 mg/5ml Susp: 300 mg/5ml Tabs: 200,300,400 mg	Neonate: 20 mg/kg/day (qid) Child: 40-60 mg/kg/day (qid/ac/qhs)
cisapride (*Propulsid*)	Tabs: 10,20 mg To make suspension crush twelve 10 mg tabs & add 12 ml propylene glycol + 18 ml NaHCO₃	0.6-1.2 mg/kg/day (tid-qid) Max dose 0.3 mg/kg If 1 mEq/1ml of NaHCO₃ is used suspension = 1mg/ml of cisapride
docusate Na⁺ (*Colace, DSS*)	Syrup: 50 & 60 mg/15ml Solution: 10&50 mg/1ml Tabs: 100 mg Caps: 50,100 ,250 mg	< 3 years: 10-40 mg (qd-qid) 3-6 years: 20-60 mg (qd-qid) 6-12 years: 40-129 mg (qd-qid)
famotidine (*Pepcid*)	Liquid: 40 mg/5 ml Tabs: 10, 20, 40 mg	1 mg/kg/day (bid-tid) Max dose 40 mg/kg/day
glycerin	infant suppository	insert + retain > 5 min (bid or qd prn)
Magic mouth-wash for gin-givostomatitis	Susp: Add *Benadryl* 30 mg + *Mylanta* 60 ml + *Carafate* 4 g	Apply small amounts to affected area prn or swish and spit. Do not exceed 5 ml *Benadryl*/day.
metoclopro-mide (*Reglan*)	Injectable: 5 mg/1ml Syrup: 5 mg/5 ml Tabs: 5,10 mg	Reflux: 0.3-0.4 mg/kg/day (tid-qid) Max dose 0.3 mg/kg
promethazine (*Phenergan*)	Supp: 12.5, 25, 50 mg Syrup: 6.25&25 mg/5ml Tabs: 12.5, 25, 50 mg	1-2 mg/kg/day (qid) (Max dose 0.5 mg/kg) **CAUTION (may mask serious illness,** only use sparingly & > 2 y)
ranitidine (*Zantac*)	Inj: 0.5 & 25 mg/1ml Syrup: 15 mg/1ml Tabs: 150, 300 mg	Prophylaxis in ICU patient: 6-8mg/kg/day (tid-qid) Ulcer: 5-10 mg/kg/day (bid-qd)
senna (*Senokot*)	Syrup: 218 mg/5 ml Tabs:187, 217, 374,600	10-20 mg/kg/dose (qhs)
sucralfate (*Carafate*)	1 gram	< 6 years: 2 g/day (qid) ≥ 6 years: 4 g/day (qid)
trimethobenz-amide (*Tigan*)	Supp: 100, 200 Caps: 100, 250	≥ 15 kg: 100-200 mg/dose tid-qid **See phenergan cautions**.

Diarrhea

Secretory diarrhea is enterotoxin-induced, (e.g., E coli, vibrio, clostridia, some staphylococcal species, shigella, salmonella). Enterotoxins cause fluid and electrolyte secretion from crypt cells and block absorption of Na^+ and Cl^- by the carrier mechanism. Glucose coupled Na^+ absorption is not blocked.

Cytotoxic diarrhea is usually due to viral agents (e.g., rotavirus) and is characterized by destruction of villous mucosa. Shortened villi decrease the intestinal surface area available for fluid absorption.

Osmotic diarrhea is usually due to malabsorption syndromes (e.g., lactose intolerance). Osmotically active agents retain fluid in the bowel lumen. Osmotic diarrhea exacerbates cytotoxic and secretory diarrhea through impaired absorption of nutrients and electrolytes. Orally administered magnesium sulfate and sorbitol cause osmotic diarrhea.

Dysenteric diarrhea is due to invasion of mucosa and submucosa of the colon and terminal ileum by infectious agents (e.g., salmonella, shigella, yersinia, campylobacter, enteroviruses). Edema, bleeding, and leukocyte infiltration typically occur.

Clinical Evaluation of the Child with Diarrhea

A bacterial origin is associated with blood in the stool in 50% of cases, and neutrophils in the stool in 70% of cases. The presence of reducing substances (measured by *Clinitest*) and a low pH suggest lactose malabsorption. Bacterial diarrheas are more common in summer. Rotavirus is the most common etiology of infectious diarrhea. Day care centers are associated with shigella, giardia, and rotavirus. Other etiologies for diarrhea include antibiotics, intussusception, gastrointestinal bleeding, and hemolytic-uremic syndrome.

Diarrhea Therapy

Oral Rehydration Therapy (ORT) is often effective, as co-transport of sodium with glucose remains intact in all types of diarrhea. World Health Organization (WHO) solution can be used in all ages (including neonates) and in those with hypotonic, isotonic, or hypertonic dehydration.

In hypernatremia, oral therapy may be superior to IV therapy. Standard glucose electrolyte solutions (e.g., *Pedialyte, Lytren*) supply electrolytes and water to correct dehydration but do not decrease stool output and have no nutritional value. Rice and wheat-based ORT are superior to standard ORT in correcting rehydration and decreasing stool output. Some clear liquids such as juices, sodas, and jello are inappropriate for treating acute diarrhea, as they contain little sodium and have high carbohydrate content which increases the osmotic load and may aggravate diarrhea (especially apple juice).

Refeeding: Gut rest is not useful. Early feeding hastens mucosal recovery and shortens the duration of illness despite increasing stool output. Breast feeding is well-tolerated. Full strength feeds are best. Some children with prolonged diarrhea develop lactose intolerance, but the majority tolerate lactose well. A BRAT diet along with wheat noodles and potatoes can be started at once. High-starch and low-fat foods are generally helpful.

Drug Therapy: Kaolin-pectin (*Kaopectate*) is an adsorbent. Bismuth subsalicylate (*PeptoBismol*) inhibits intestinal secretions and is useful in traveler's diarrhea. Antibiotics are indicated for shigella, vibrio cholera, and enteroinvasive E coli. Sulfamethoxazole/trimethoprim (*Septra* or *Bactrim*) is the drug of choice for shigella, vibrio, and E coli. Antibiotics for salmonella are indicated if < 3-6 months old, or immunocompromised patients. Erythromycin is effective for campylobacter. See page 64 for antibiotic recommendations and dosing.

Chronic diarrhea: Culture the stool and test for lactose intolerance (reducing substances and low pH). If lactose intolerance suspected, discontinue dairy products for 2 weeks.

Discharge instructions for diarrhea
- Administer clear liquids such as *Pedialyte, Lytren,* and *Ricelyte* in smaller children. Older children may be given *Gatorade, Jell-O* water or diluted cola. Do not give plain water or juices. If no vomiting, administer large amounts of fluid every 3-4 hours. If vomiting, give small sips every 10-15 minutes; slowly increase amount and decrease frequency of feeding.
- Start refeeding in 8 to 24 hours even if diarrhea is present. In an infant, start with full-strength regular formula. If the diarrhea is prolonged or worsens after administration of lactose-based formula switch to a soy-based formula.
- If child tolerates solids, give a BRAT diet (bananas, rice, applesauce, toast) and noodles or potatoes.
- Physician reevaluation if bloody stool, bilious vomiting, or worsened symptoms.

Upper Gastrointestinal Bleeding - Etiology

Age	Most Frequent Cause	Features
0-30 days	• Ingested maternal blood • Bleeding diathesis • Gastric ulcers • Gastritis, esophagitis,	See Apt Downey test See below[1] Premature, other stressors
> 30 days – 2 years	• Stress ulcers • Gastritis, esophagitis, Mallory Weiss tears (MW)	
2-6 years	• Gastric ulcer, gastritis, varices • Esophagitis, MW, hemophilia	Varices occur with liver disease primarily
> 6 years	• Peptic ulcer, gastritis, • Esophagitis (due to reflux, chemicals or infection)	

[1] Hemorrhagic disease of newborn or aspirin, phenytoin, phenobarbital, promethazine, cephalothin

Lower Gastrointestinal Bleeding – Etiology

Age	Most Frequent Cause	Features
0-30 days	• Maternal blood, anal fissure • Bleeding diathesis • Infectious, allergic colitis • Necrotizing enterocolitis • Volvulus, Hirschsprung's	See Apt Downey test Allergy to milk/soy protein Esp. premature < 2 weeks
> 30 days – 2 years	• Anal fissure, infectious • Intussusception, Meckel's • Milk allergy, juvenile polyps • Intestinal duplication, hemolytic uremic syndrome (HUS)	See page 89, 90 See page 76 See page 55
2-6 years	• Infectious • Juvenile polyps • Anal fissure, intussusception • Meckel's, inflammatory bowel • Henoch Schonlein Purpura (HSP)	Painless, bright blood See intussusception below See Meckel's scan below See page 55
> 6 years	• Inflammatory bowel disease • Infectious, juvenile polyps • HUS, HSP, hemorrhoids	See pages 55

Evaluation and Management of GI Bleeding

- Place cardiac monitor, administer O_2, and insert at least two large bore IV's.
- Draw CBC, clotting studies, type and cross at least 15 ml/kg of packed RBC's.
- Administer 20 ml/kg NS bolus and repeat to correct hypotension or shock.
- Consider transfusion if there is no response to first two fluid boluses.
- **Endoscopy** identifies bleeding site in 75-90% of upper GI bleeding.
- **Urgent surgery** indications: unrelenting hemorrhage, > 50-75 ml/kg blood transfused in 2 hours, perforation, or vascular compromise.
- **Contrast studies** are not indicated acutely. Angiography will only detect a bleeding site if the bleeding rate is > 0.5-2.0 ml/minute.
- **Radionuclide scanning** (Tc99) may detect low grade GI bleeding from a Meckel's diverticulum. Tc99 has an affinity for parietal cells present in gastric mucosa and in 90% of Meckel's diverticulum. A positive scan consists of a persistent focus of uptake in the right lower quadrant or lower abdomen. This test is indicated for any child < 3 years old who presents with painless lower GI bleeding. This test is 85% sensitive and 92% specific for Meckel's.

Erroneous Stool Guaiac Testing: Acidic pH lowers the sensitivity of guaiac, so use specific gastric test cards (e.g., *Gastroccult*) when evaluating for upper GI bleed.
- *False positive:* Iron, red fruits, meats, iodine, bromide, or chlorophyll
- *False negative:* Dried stool specimens, vitamin C or certain antacids

Apt-Downey Test for Fetal vs. Maternal Blood: Mix stool in a test tube with an equal quantity of tap water. Centrifuge or filter out solids. Add one part 1.0% NaOH to five parts of supernatant. Read in 2 minutes. Fetal Hb resists alkali denaturation. A persistent pink color indicates the presence of fetal Hb. If supernatant turns yellow, Hb is adult and thus maternal.

Neonatal - Jaundice

Newborns exhibit hepatic insufficiency that resolves within 1st 4-6 weeks. The 50th percentile for bilirubin in normal neonates is 6 mg/dl (6% have levels > 12 mg/dl) Jaundice is usually noted at 5 mg/dl in infants and 2 mg/dl if older. Hyperbilirubinemia is associated with breast feeding, weight loss, maternal diabetes, Asian race, oxytocin, ↓gestational age, and male sex. Prolonged unconjugated hyperbilirubinemia can lead to kernicterus. Precise level of bilirubin that is toxic for an individual infant is unknown. Early signs of kernicterus: lethargy, poor feeding, loss of Moro reflex, seizures and movement disorders (late sign). Direct bilirubin should be ≤ 15% of total (conjugated + unconjugated or direct + indirect). Conjugated hyperbilirubinemia is abnormal and should always provoke further evaluation.

Hyperbilirubinemia Management for Healthy Term Newborns

Age (if < 24 hours old see below)	25-48 hrs	49-72 hrs	> 72 hrs
	Total serum bilirubin in mg/dl (μmol/L)		
Consider Phototherapy	≥ 12 (170)	≥ 15 (260)	≥ 17 (290)
Phototherapy	≥ 15 (260)	≥ 18 (310)	≥ 20 (340)
Exchange Therapy if Phototherapy Fails	≥ 20 (340)	≥ 25 (430)	≥ 25 (430)
Exchange Therapy and Phototherapy	≥ 25 (430)	≥ 30 (510)	≥ 30 (510)

(*Pediatrics* 1994;565)

Factors Associated with Non-physiologic Jaundice

- Jaundice in infant < 24 hours old or non-breastfed infant > 1 week old
- Serum bilirubin rise of > 5 mg/dl/day or > 0.5 mg/dl/hour
- Serum bilirubin > 15 mg/dl in a full term neonate (lower if premature)
- Jaundice persisting > 1 week in a full term or more than 2 weeks if postterm
- Conjugated ↑ bili (e.g., obstruction, infection, toxin/drugs or metabolic/genetic)
- Ill appearance, infection or GI obstruction suspected, or abnormal labs below

Evaluation of Neonatal Jaundice

Recommended Lab tests	Direct/indirect bilirubin, CBC/differential, retic. count & peripheral smear, Coomb's test (if mother's blood type unknown)
If >1 week old add	Liver and thyroid function tests
Consider	Work-ups for sepsis & TORCH, evaluation for GI obstruction

Treatment of Hyperbilirubinemia

- Exchange transfusion if bilirubin > 20-25 mg/dl in a term neonate, or at lower level in premature neonate (exact level controversial)
- Phototherapy if within 5 mg/dl of exchange transfusion level
- Phototherapy if there is an ↑ total serum bilirubin of > 1-2 mg/dl in 4-6 hours
- Perform exchange transfusion at lower levels if signs of kernicterus are present
- Treat underlying disorder (e.g. sepsis, GI tract obstruction)

Anemia

Normal RBC Indices (mean ± 2 standard deviations)

Age	Hb(g/dl)	Hct(%)	MCV(fl)	MCH(pg)	MCHC(g/dl)
Birth	16.5 ± 3.0	51 ± 9	108 ± 10	34 ± 3	33 ± 3
1-3 days	18.5 ± 4.0	56 ± 14	108 ± 13	34 ± 3	33 ± 4
1 week	17.5 ± 4.0	54 ± 12	107 ± 19	34 ± 6	33 ± 5
2 weeks	16.5 ± 4.0	51 ± 12	105 ± 19	34 ± 6	33 ± 5
1 month	14.0 ± 4.0	43 ± 12	104 ± 19	34 ± 6	33 ± 4
2 months	11.5 ± 2.5	35 ± 7	96 ± 19	30 ± 4	33 ± 4
3-6 months	11.5 ± 2.0	35 ± 6	91 ± 17	30 ± 5	33 ± 3
0.5-2 years	12.0 ± 1.5	36 ± 3	78 ± 8	27 ± 4	33 ± 3
2-6 years	12.5 ± 1.0	37 ± 3	81 ± 6	27 ± 3	34 ± 3
6-12 years	13.5 ± 2.0	40 ± 5	86 ± 9	29 ± 4	34 ± 3
12-18y female	14.0 ± 2.0	41 ± 5	90 ± 12	30 ± 5	34 ± 3
12-18y male	14.5 ± 1.5	43 ± 6	88 ± 10	30 ± 5	34 ± 3

Causes of Anemia by Age

Neonate: Blood loss, isoimmunization or congenital hemolytic anemia

3-6 months: Congenital disorder of hemoglobin synthesis (e.g., thalassemia)

6 months to 2 years: Iron deficiency is associated with early or excessive cow's milk. Hereditary hemolytic anemia (spherocytosis, hemoglobinopathy, or red cell enzyme deficiency) suggested by a family history of anemia, jaundice, gallstones or splenectomy. B_{12} deficiency suggested by tortuous retinal vessels (hemoglobinopathy), glossitis and diminished vibratory/position sense. RBC distribution width (RDW) reflects cell heterogeneity. Variable RDW sizes are seen in hemolysis or reticulocytosis. Markedly high WBC counts, high glucose, sodium, and triglycerides falsely elevate RBC counts.

Anemia Differential Diagnosis

Microcytic	Iron deficiency (RDW > 14%), thalassemia (RDW < 14%), chronic inflammation, sideroblastic anemia, lead poisoning, B_6 deficiency
Macrocytic	Folic acid or B_{12} deficiency, Fanconi's, hepatic disease
Normocytic (high retics)	*Extrinsic disorders*: antibody-mediated hemolysis, fragmentation hemolysis, DIC, hemolytic uremic syndrome, artificial heart valves, liver and renal disease. *Intrinsic disorders*: membrane disorders (spherocytosis, elliptocytosis), enzyme deficiencies (glucose-6-phosphate dehydrogenase or pyruvate kinase deficiency), hemoglobin disorders (SS, SC, S-thalassemia).
Normocytic (low retics)	Diamond Blackfan, transient erythroblastopenia of childhood, aplastic crisis, bone marrow infiltrate (leukemia, metastatic disease), renal disease, infection, malnutrition

---

Sickle Cell Anemia

Diagnosis and evaluation of patients with sickle cell disease

- Sickle cell screen may be negative up to 4-6 months of age and in sickle trait.
- A routine Hb is recommended to assess severity or change of anemia.
- Consider a reticulocyte count to screen for aplastic crisis (Mean reticulocyte for sickle cell patient is 12%, in aplastic crises it may be <3%).
- Urine specific gravity is not a useful test for dehydration, as it may be low from isosthenuria (inability to concentrate the urine).

Fever in Sickle Cell Anemia

Penicillin prophylaxis decreases the incidence of sepsis and death for sickle cell children aged 6 months to 5 years. As a rule, febrile children with sickle cell disease are admitted and treated with IV antibiotics. However, recent criteria have been published that define a subset of patients that may be treated as outpatients.

Criteria for Outpatient Management of Fever in Sickle Cell Patients

• Yale observation score < 10 (pg 66)	• WBC count > 5,000 and < 30,000
• Normal blood pressure	• Hb > 5 g/dl, Platelets > 100,000
• No prior pneumococcal sepsis	• Administer ceftriaxone 50 mg/kg
• Mild pain only	IV/IM if no allergy to cephalosporin
• No pneumonia	• Reliable 24 hour follow up with
• Normal capillary refill	repeat ceftriaxone dose in 24 hours
• Temperature < 40°C (104°F)	

Wilimas. *New Engl J Med* 1993; 329: 472

Management of Sickle Cell Disease Complications

Painful crises (all ages)

> Most common sites of pain in order of decreasing frequency: Lumbosacral spine, thigh and hip, knee, abdomen, shoulder, chest. Intravenous morphine is the treatment of choice, and should be titrated. Meperidine is not recommended (especially in high or repeated doses), as a metabolite (normeperidine) can cause CNS excitation and seizures. Hydration (oral or IV) and oxygen are commonly accepted adjunctive therapy.

Splenic sequestration crisis (1 - 6 years)

> Associated with an acute drop of Hb >3 g/dl or total Hb <6 g/dl. Due to splenic vein vaso-occlusion. Abdominal pain, shock, and hypotension may occur. Second only to sepsis as cause of death in children with sickle cell. Patients are usually < 6 years old (if have SS disease) but older if have SC or S-B-thalassemia variants. Patients present with sudden hypovolemic shock or a slow increase in spleen size. Obtain CBC, type and cross, and reticulocyte count. Admit and treat hypovolemia.

Management of Sickle Cell Disease Complications

Acute chest syndrome (all ages)

    The complex of pulmonary symptoms and a pulmonary infiltrate in a patient with sickle cell disease. Admit and rule out pulmonary embolus. Antibiotic therapy for pneumonia is recommended (e.g., erythromycin and cefuroxime).

Hand foot syndrome (dactylitis, 6 months to 6 years)

    Due to vaso-occlusion in the hands and feet. This is the most common presentation of sickle cell anemia at 6-24 months, and often the first crisis experienced. Nonpitting edema from symmetric infarction of the metacarpals/metatarsals occurs. Treat as a pain crisis.

Sickle stroke (all ages)

    Occurs in 10-20% of children with sickle cell disease. Mean age is 10 years. Strokes are usually ischemic, although hemorrhagic strokes may occur in older children. Treat by exchange transfusion to keep hemoglobin S < 20% of total.

Aplastic crisis (6 months to young adulthood)

    Parvovirus is the most common identified precipitant. Other common causes include drug toxicity (phenylbutazone) and folate deficiency. Hallmark is reticulocyte count < 3%. Transfuse these patients if they are severely anemic.

Cardiac complications

    Patients may develop congestive heart failure.

Abdominal complications

    Liver, splenic and mesenteric infarctions may occur. Bilirubin gallstones are common although < 10% are symptomatic.

Genitourinary complications

    Priapism may develop. Priapism lasting > 3 hours is unlikely to resolve spontaneously. Treatment of priapism consists of hydration, oxygen, pain management, and possibly exchange transfusion. These patients are less likely to require surgery to correct priapism than patients without sickle cell disease. Additionally, painless hematuria and renal papillary necrosis may occur, and isosthenuria (difficulty concentrating urine) may develop.

Bone complications

    Avascular necrosis of the femoral head occurs in 12% of patients. Sickle dactylitis can cause small lytic lesions in the digits.

Causes of Abnormal Bleeding Tests[1]

Lab Value	Causes
thrombocytopenia ↓platelet count (<150,000/ml)	Decreased production of platelets (due to drugs, toxins or infections), splenic sequestration or platelet pooling, platelet destruction (due to collagen vascular disease, drugs, post transfusion, infection, ITP, DIC, TTP, HUS, or vasculitis)
platelet dysfunction (with normal count)	Adhesion defects (e.g., von Willibrand's disease) or aggregation defects (e.g., thrombasthenia)
↑BT (>9 minutes)	All platelet disorders, DIC, ITP, uremia, liver failure, aspirin
↑PTT (>35 sec)	Coagulation pathway defects (common factors 2, 5, 10, intrinsic 8, 9, 11, 12), DIC, liver failure, heparin
↑PT (>12-13 sec)	Coagulation pathway defects (common factors 2, 5, 10, extrinsic 7) DIC, liver failure, warfarin
↑TT (>8-10 sec)	DIC, liver failure or uremia, heparin
↓ fibrinogen, ↑FSP	ITP, liver failure

[1] BT-bleeding time, TT-Thrombin time, PTT-partial thromboplastin time, PT-prothrombin time, DIC-disseminated intravascular coagulopathy, ITP-idiopathic thrombocytopenic purpura, TTP-thrombotic thrombocytopenic purpura, HUS-hemolytic uremic syndrome.

Platelet and capillary disorders cause mucous membrane bleeds (GI, epistaxis, prolonged bleed with cuts, petechiae (↑bleeding time and abnormal platelets).
Coagulation disorders cause deep muscle + CNS bleeds, hemarthrosis, ↑PT/PTT.

Dosing of Replacement Factors

Medication	Dose
Factor VIII	• [desired activity level (%) – baseline activity level (%)] ÷2 • 1 unit/kg factor 8↑activity level 2% (factor 8 T½ = 12 hours)[1]
Factor IX	• desired activity level (%) - baseline activity level (%) • 1 unit/kg factor 9↑activity level 1% (factor 9 T½ = 24 hours) [1]
DDAVP *Desmo-pressin*	• 0.3 µg/kg in 50 ml NS IV over 30 minutes • possibly effective via nasal spray or SC injection, recommended only if baseline activity > 10%

[1] T½ = half life

Factor Replacements

Product	Forms	Contents	Units/bag[1]
cryopre-cipitate	cryoprecipitate	factor VII, vWf [2] fibrinogen,	100
factor VIII	*Recombinate, Bioclate, Kogenate* (all recombinant factor 8)	factor VIII, human albumin	250,500, 1000
factor IX	*Konyne, Feiba, Alphanine, Proplex, Autoplex,* prothrombin concentrates	factors II, VIII, IX, X	400-600

[1] Units/bag should be indicated on the label. [2] von Willebrand factor

Factor VIII Deficiency Treatment

Bleed type	%Activity Desired	Dose[1] (units/kg)	Duration of Therapy
Severe[1]			
CNS injury	80-100%	50	14 days
GI bleed	80-100%	50	3 days more than bleed
Major trauma	80-100%	50	depends on injuries
Retroperitoneal	80-100%	50	6 days
Retropharyngeal	80-100%	50	4 days
Pending surgery	80-100%	50	variable
Moderate[2]			
Mild head trauma	50%	25	variable
Deep muscle	50%	25	q day until resolution
Hip or groin injury	40%	20	repeat once in 1-2 days
Mouth, lip, dental[3]	40%	20	variable
Hematuria[4]	40%	20	3-5 days
Mild[2]			
Laceration	20%	10	until sutures out for 24h
Common joint	20-40%	10-20	recheck in 1-2 days
Soft tissue / Small muscle[5]	20-40%	10-20	variable

[1] If baseline activity is 0%. Assume all severe bleeding cases have baseline of 0%.

[2] Desmopressin (DDAVP) 0.3 μg/kg IV or intranasal or subcutaneous has been used for mild and moderate bleeding states, especially useful if baseline factor is > 10%.

[3] To prepare for dental/oropharyngeal procedures, consider aminocaproic acid (*Amicar*) 100 mg/kg PO q6h for 6 days or cyclokapron 25 mg/kg q6h for 6 days. Also consider topical epinephrine, *Surgicel*, or *Avitene*. CAUTERY MAY WORSEN BLEEDING.

[4] Consider prednisone (2 mg/kg/day x 2d) and oral fluids without factor replacement if mild.

[5] Consider admission to observe for compartment syndrome.

- Epistaxis and minor lacerations may not need replacement.

- Recommended dosing is variable, and if the situation allows contact the patient's hematologist for verification of actual doses.

Inhibitors: Patients with inhibitors may have poor response to factor VIII. Inhibitor level to factor 8 is measured by Bethesda Unit Titer (BUT). To determine therapy you must know the bleeding severity, inhibitor level, and prior response to transfused factor VIII. High responders have marked increase inhibitor levels ~ 5 d after factor VIII infusion. Factor VIII may be used to treat if low titer inhibitor (<2 BUT). Factor IX at 50-100 units/kg may be used for minor bleeds. If significant bleeding, massive doses of factor VIII may be effective. If high titer of inhibitor (>10 BUT) and activated factor IX concentrates (*Feiba* or *Autoplex* are not successful...

patients may benefit from plasmaphoresis and factor replacement of porcine factor concentrate. If activity > 5-10%, mix desmopressin _(DDAVP)_ with NS and infuse over 30 min at 0.3 µg/kg q48h. This is useful in von Willebrand's disease, but may cause seizures and hyponatremia in children < 4 years old.

Fresh frozen plasma (FFP) contains all coagulation factors and can be used for unknown bleeding disorders. FFP or cryoprecipitate can be used to treat von Willebrand's disease. FFP 40 ml/kg will raise blood activity of any factor to 100%, however, this high volume may cause fluid overload in certain patients.

Cryoprecipitate contains 5-10 units of factor 8 activity per ml (1 bag contains 10 ml or 50-100 units of factor 8 activity).

Desmopressin (DDAVP) dose is 0.3 µg/kg IV, and can be used for mild to moderate bleeding in von Willebrand's disease and hemophilia A.

Prothrombin complex (factors 2, 7, 9, 10) can be used to treat hemophilia B but can precipitate thrombi and/or disseminated intravascular coagulation (DIC).

Blood Products and Transfusion (see page 54 for dosing)

Crossmatching and ordering blood products: Type-specific non-crossmatched blood causes a fatality in 1 in 30 million transfusions. Non-ABO antibodies occur in 0.04% of non-transfused and 0.3% of previously transfused.

Whole blood has no WBC's and 20% of normal platelets after 24 h storage. Factors V + VIII decline to 40% after 21 d. 70% of RBC's remain after 21-35 d storage. With storage, K^+ & ammonia increase (beware in liver failure) and Ca^{+2} decreases (beware in liver dysfunction as citrate is not effectively metabolized by the liver).

Packed Red Blood Cells (PRBC's): Hematocrit rises 1% for each ml/kg of PRBC's transfused. Fewer antigens are present in PRBC's compared to whole blood. (1) _Leukocyte poor RBC's_ are derived from filtering RBC's and should be used if one severe, or 2 sequential febrile non-hemolytic transfusion reactions. (2) _Washed RBC's_ are useful in patients with prior anaphylaxis due to antibodies to IgA or other proteins. (3) _Frozen deglycerolized RBC's_ are the purest RBC product. Use if there is a reaction to washed RBC's or a transfusion reaction due to Anti-IgA antibodies.

Fresh frozen plasma (FFP) ABO cross-match prior to transfusion. Indications: (1) coagulation protein deficiency when specific factor concentrates are undesirable or unavailable, (2) _Coumadin_ reversal, (3) diffuse bleeding + documented coagulopathy, or (4) active bleeding with liver disease and a secondary coagulopathy.

Factor VIII preparations: (1) cryoprecipitate is made from single donor and contains fibrinogen, von Willebrand's factor, and factors 8 and 13 (2) factor 8 concentrate is pooled from multiple donors (3) several recombinant factor 8 products are available.

Factor IX concentrate: Prothrombin complex contains factors II, VII, IX, and X. One unit raises a recipient's activity 1.5%. Factors IX and X are thrombogenic and can cause DIC; therefore, use cautiously in hepatic and vascular disease.

Platelet concentrate: One unit = 5-10 thousand platelets. Platelets are not refrigerated and only survive 7 days. Platelet counts > 50,000/ml are desirable prior to surgery. ABO cross-matching is not necessary.

Albumin and plasma protein fraction (PPF): 25% salt-poor albumin contains excess sodium (160 mEq Na+/L) and is hyperoncotic compared to plasma. 5% buffered albumin solution is iso-oncotic compared to plasma. PPF contains 88% albumin and 12% globulins and is iso-oncotic compared to plasma.

Testing Blood Prior to Administration

Complete crossmatch - 3 phases (1) Immediate spin phase detects ABO-incompatibility from IgM and takes 5-10 min. (2) Albumin phase takes 15-30 min. (3) Antihuman globulin phase takes 15-30 min. Albumin and antihuman globulin phases detect IgM, IgG, + other antibodies causing hemolytic transfusion reactions.

Unexpected antibody screen uncovers non ABO antibodies (e.g. Kell, Duffy) in recipient's serum. 0.04% of recipients will have a unexpected + antibody screen if no prior transfusion, and 1% will have a positive screen if prior transfusion. This test is important if prior transfusion or pregnancy.

Abbreviated crossmatch: (1) immediate spin alone, or (2) stat crossmatch - omit immediate spin and shorten antihuman globulin and albumin phase to 15 minutes.

Transfusion Reactions

Hemolytic transfusion reactions occur in 1/40,000 transfusions and are usually due to ABO incompatibility. Symptoms: palpitations, abdominal and back pain, syncope, and sensation of doom. Consider if temperature rises ≥ 2C. Immediately stop transfusion, and look for hemoglobinemia and hemoglobinuria. Perform direct antiglobulin (Coomb's test), haptoglobin, peripheral smear, serum bilirubin, and repeat antibody screen + crossmatch. Keep urine output ≥ 100 ml/hour and consider alkalization of urine to limit renal failure. Mannitol is not useful; it increases urine flow by decreasing tubular reabsorption without improving renal perfusion.

Anaphylactic reaction almost exclusively occurs with Anti-IgA antibodies (1/70 people). It usually begins after the first few ml of blood with afebrile flushing, wheezing, cramps, vomiting, diarrhea, and hypotension. Discontinue the transfusion and treat with diphenhydramine, epinephrine and steroids.

Febrile non-hemolytic reactions occur during or soon after initiation of 3-4% of all transfusions, most frequently in multiply transfused or multiparous patients with antileukocyte antibodies. Stop transfusion and treat as transfusion reaction.

Urticarial reactions cause local erythema, hives and itching. Further evaluation unnecessary unless fever, chills, or other adverse effects are present. This is the only type of transfusion reaction in which the infusion can continue.

Infections: AIDS, CMV, or hepatitis may be transmitted with blood products

Blood Products

Component	Indication	Dose	Adverse effects	Special Features
albumin 5%[1]	shock	10-20 ml/kg	rare volume overload, fever, urticaria	stable storage, no filter needed, no disease transmission
PPF (Plasmanate)[1]	same as above	10-20 ml/kg	above and hypotension	above
hetastarch 6% (Hespan)[1]	volume expansion	10-20 ml/kg	pruritis, coagulopathy	stable leukopheresis, no disease transmission
Dextran 40[1]	volume expansion	10 ml/kg	anaphylaxis, bleeding	same as hetastarch
Dextran 70[1]	volume expansion	10 ml/kg	above and renal failure	same as hetastarch
whole blood[2]	hemorrhagic shock	10 ml/kg ↑ Hb 1g/dl	transfusion reactions, hemolysis, disease transmission	thrombocytopenia, coagulopathy, leukopenia
packed RBC's[2]	↑O_2 carrying capacity	3 ml/kg ↑ Hb 1g/dl	less allergic and febrile reactions than whole blood	same as whole blood; hematocrit is 70-80%, dilute in 0.9 NS due to viscosity
washed RBC's	↓ allergic reactions	" "	rare	takes 1 hour to wash and >70% of RBC's lost
leukocyte poor RBC's	99.9% of WBC's are removed	" "	rare	use if two prior febrile non-hemolytic reactions to washed RBC's
platelet concentrate	poorly functioning or decreased platelets	1 unit/10 kg	transfusion reactions are rare	no cross-matching needed, but ABO blood group compatibility is preferred
FFP (fresh frozen plasma)	coagulopathy with bleed	10-20 ml/kg	transfusion reactions are rare	no cross-matching needed, but ABO blood group compatibility is preferred

[1]No cross-match needed. [2]For acute hemorrhage, initiate transfusion with 20 ml/kg of whole blood or 10 ml/kg of PRBC's. No medications can be added to any blood component. Request sickle prep negative blood for sickle cell patients. Avoid mixing blood with D5W and Ringer's lactate because of hemolysis and clotting, respectively.

Hemolytic Uremic Syndrome (HUS)

HUS - a post-infectious disorder causing (1) nephropathy, (2) microangiopathic hemolytic anemia, & (3) thrombocytopenia. It commonly occurs < 5 years old following a URI or gastroenteritis (esp. E. coli 0157:H7, *Shigella, Salmonella*). Organisms produce toxin that kills GI organ cells. 30% reoccur. **Treatment:** Manage complications: uremia (dialysis), anti-hypertensives (if↑BP), fluids & blood (bleed or↓BP), anti-seizures prn, platelets prn. *Dialyze* if (1) congestive heart failure (2) BUN > 100 mg/dl, (3) encephalopathy, (4) anuria > 24 hours (5) ↑K⁺

Clinical Features
• *Prodome* - URI or gastroenteritis
• *GI* – 75% have pain (can cause intussusception, or perforation), vomiting, or diarrhea (often bloody)
• ↓*Urination* (gross hematuria rare)
• *Skin* – pallor, petechiae, purpura
• *Hypertension* (in up to 50%)
• *CNS*- seizure, coma, encephalopathy

Laboratory Features
• Urine – hematuria, proteinuria, casts
• CBC – ↓Hb, ↓ platelets, ↓WBC
• Smear – schistocytes, helmet cells
• ↓Na⁺, ↓CO₂, ↑K⁺, ↑BUN, ↑creatinine
• PT/PTT are usually normal

Henoch-Schonlein Purpura

Overview HSP is a systemic vasculitis with skin, joint, GI, or renal involvement. Scrotal, CNS, heart, and lung involvement are less common. HSP without skin involvement is called *HSP syndrome*. HSP peaks at 4-5 years, but can occur at any age. It is more common in winter & early spring. Precipitants: streptococci, mycoplasma, hepatitis B, salicylates, antibiotics, and food allergens. HSP is pathophysiologically a small vessel vasculitis, with WBC's infiltrating and necrosing the walls of capillaries, arterioles, and venules. **Treatment** Supportive care and steroids are used for abdominal pain and renal involvement, although their benefit has not been clearly established.

Clinical features
• *Skin* – involved in most. Petechiae, coalesce to large ecchymoses. Purpura are gravity dependent occurring on the buttock and legs.
• *Painless edema* – 25-35% (usually at dorsum of hands and feet), with painful edema of face, scalp.
• *GI tract* – 50-90% with vomiting, or bleeding. Intussusception (3-6%), pancreatitis, or bowel infarcts occur.
• *Joint* involvement in 50-75% usually knees/ankles, transitory periarticular swelling, non-migratory. This is 1st site in 25% & resolves with rest
• *Renal* - 50% and may be the only site that is permanent. Episodic gross hematuria occurs in 30-40%.

Hypertension

Hypertensive encephalopathy is the most common presentation of acute hypertension (HTN), with headache, confusion, vomiting, and/or focal neurologic findings. Severe HTN is defined as a systolic BP above the 99th percentile for a given age or >15 mmHg above the 95th percentile. Malignant HTN is severe HTN with retinal changes, papilledema, and widespread fibrinoid necrosis of arterioles.

	Age	Systolic BP	Diastolic BP
Age-Based Definition of "Severe" Hypertension:	Newborn-7 days	$\geq$106	--
	1-2 years	$\geq$118	$\geq$82
	3-5 years	$\geq$124	$\geq$84
(Task force on BP in children, Pediatrics 1987; 79:1)	6-9 years	$\geq$130	$\geq$86
	10-12 years	$\geq$134	$\geq$90
	13-15 years	$\geq$144	$\geq$92
	16-18 years	$\geq$150	$\geq$98

Etiology of Pediatric Hypertension (HTN)

- *Renal disease* is the most common cause of both acute and chronic HTN. HTN and encephalopathy (or seizures) may be the initial presentation of acute post-streptococcal glomerulonephritis. Sodium retention and volume expansion occur due to diminished glomerular filtration rate, resulting in an acute rise in BP. Findings in nephritis include hematuria, periorbital edema, & RBC casts.

- *CNS disease*: Cushing's triad of bradycardia, bradypnea, and HTN are found with increased intracranial pressure, and can result from intracerebral tumors, hemorrhage, trauma, or infection.

- *Neuroblastomas* can cause HTN due to increased catecholamine release, similar to neurofibromatosis and pheochromocytoma. This HTN may be episodic, and associated with flushing, palpitations, anxiety, sweating, and chest pain. Cortical adrenal tumors secrete cortisol and can cause HTN.

- *Drug toxicity*: HTN can be due to various mechanisms from steroids, non-steroidal anti-inflammatories, phenylephrine, pseudoephedrine, albuterol, cyclosporine A, and drugs of abuse. Chronic lead toxicity can cause HTN, as can licorice through its mineralocorticoid effects.

- *Aortic coarctation* (CoA) is the most common cause of HTN in the first year of life. CoA also causes up to 2% of secondary HTN in children and adolescents.

- *Other*: Burn victims often exhibit HTN due to sympathetic discharge. 43% of babies with bronchopulmonary dysplasia exhibit HTN.

Drugs in Hypertensive Emergencies *(Pediatr Ann 1996; 25:368; Pediatr EM Rep 1998; 3:39)*

Drug	Dose (max), route, preparation	Mechanism	Onset (Duration)	Features
captopril (Capoten)	test dose: 0.01 mg/kg PO, then 0.15-0.2 mg/kg PO, double q 2 h until BP control. (max: 4-6 mg/kg/day - bid-tid) Tabs: 12.5, 25, 50, 100 mg	ACE inhibitor	15 min (12h)	useful in renin-induced HTN, side effects include dry cough, rash, angioedema, neutropenia, proteinuria, ↑ K+ and creatinine
enalapril (Vasotec)	0.05-0.1 mg/kg/day (max: 0.5 mg/kg/day) (give qd or bid) Tabs: 2.5, 5, 10, 20 mg	ACE inhibitor	1 h (6 h)	see captopril: consider test dose of 0.01 mg/kg if no prior use
esmolol (Brevibloc)	500 µg/kg IV over 1st min, then titrate 50-200 µg/kg/min	β-blockade	sec (9min)	can cause or worsen bronchospasm, bradycardia
fenoldopam mesylate (Corlopam)	0.1-2.0 µg/kg/min IV infusion	Dopamine-1 receptor agonist	4 min (10 min)	↑ renal flow, & Na+ excretion, contains metabisifite (allergy)
furosemide (Lasix)	1.4 mg/kg IV	loop diuretic	5 min (3h)	hyperglycemia
labatalol (Normodyne)	Start at 0.2 mg/kg IV; double dose q15 min pm (max: 2-3 mg/kg/dose)	α + β blockade in 1:7 ratio	sec (6h)	bronchospasm
nicardipine (Cardene)	0.03mg/kg IV or 1-5 µg /kg/min IV	Ca channel block	2 min (40 min)	↑ ICP, ↑HR, ↑V/Q mismatch
nifedipine (Procardia)	0.25-0.50 mg/kg PO/SL or max: 1mg/kg/day Caps: 10,20 mg; Tabs: 30,60,90 mg	Ca channel blocker	2 min (6h)	may ↑ ICP, facial flushing, may too rapidly lower pressure causing stroke, or hypoperfusion
nimodipine (Nimotop)	0.35 mg/kg PO (max: 30-60 mg/dose q4-6) Tabs: 30 mg	Ca channel blocker	1 h (9h)	not approved < 12 yr, ↓ neuro deficit in subarachnoid bleed
propranolol (Inderal)	0.01-0.1 mg/kg IV over 10min (max: 1 mg)	β-blockade	sec (8h)	bradycardia, bronchospasm
sodium nitroprusside (Nipride)	0.5-8 µg/kg/min IV infusion	arterial and venous dilator	sec (min)	no↓cardiac output, possible cyanide toxicity and ↑ ICP

sec-seconds, min-minutes, h-hours, mo-months, mg-milligrams, µg-micrograms, IV-intravenous, PO-oral, SL-sublingual, IM-intramuscular

Hypertensive Encephalopathy

BP autoregulation is lost and vasodilation occurs causing cerebral ischemia. Vasodilators in children with HTN and ↑ ICP may be detrimental. Patients with underlying chronic HTN are less likely to develop acute symptoms. Search for underlying disease and end-organ damage in any patient with acute HTN.

Treatment of Hypertensive Encephalopathy (see page 57 for dosing)

- <u>Sodium nitroprusside</u> (*Nipride*) by IV infusion is the drug of choice, due to its rapid onset and short half-life. It is light sensitive. Metabolism produces cyanide which is detoxified to thiocyanate and renally excreted. Nitroprusside also causes cerebral vasodilation and may theoretically increase intracranial pressure. This is the drug of choice for most hypertensive emergencies unless there is a space occupying cranial lesion or significant renal failure.
- <u>Nicardipine</u> is extremely effective for controlled reduction of BP in children and the 2nd most common agent recommended for hypertensive emergencies. It ↓peripheral vascular resistance, has little effect on heart rate and can↑ICP.
- <u>Labetolol</u> (*Normodyne*) is an $\alpha + \beta$ blocker. It is relatively safe in patients with renal disease and metabolized by the liver. This agent does not ↑ ICP. It is less potent than nicardipine, and *Nipride*, produces a reduction in cardiac output, and may cause bronchospasm and worsen congestive heart failure.
- <u>Nifedipine</u> Recent studies recommend **caution** with this drug due to uncontrolled BP lowering effects producing cerebral or coronary ischemia.
- <u>Fenoldopam</u> (*Corlopam*) dopamine 1 receptor agonist. Titratable IV with good safety profile

---

Immunizations

CHILDHOOD IMMUNIZATION SCHEDULE				Months				Years		
Age	Birth	2	4	6	12	15	18	4-6	11-12	14-16
Hepatitis B	HB-1									
			HB-2		HB-3					
DTP*		DTP	DTP	DTP		DTP		DTP	dT	
H influenza b		Hib	Hib	Hib	Hib					
Polio†		OPV	OPV		OPV			OPV		
MMR					MMR			MMR		
Varicella					Varicella					

* Acellular pertussis form preferred for all DTP doses, but whole cell is acceptable.
† Inactivated polio vacine (IPV) an alternative for either first 2 or all doses.

Hepatitis B Exposure

Type of exposure	Status of source is	Treatment if exposed patient is	
		Unvaccinated	Vaccinated
percutaneous or mucosal	HBsAg +	HBIG, HBV	HBV & HBIG if exposed HBsAb -
known source	high risk for HBsAg +	HBV and HBIG if source HBsAg +	HBV & HBIG if source HBsAg+ & exposed HBsAb-
known source	low HbsAg+ ris	HBV	none
unknown	unknown	HBV	none
sex / perinatal	HBsAg +	HBIG, HBV	none
house/work	HBsAg +	none	none

HBIG = hepatitis B immune globulin. Dose 0.06 ml/kg IM or 0.5 ml total if perinatal.
HBV = hepatitis B vaccine. Dose 20 µg/kg IM in deltoid initially, repeat in 1 & 6 mo.
Hepatitis C exposure: ± Administer immune serum globulin (ISG) 0.06 ml/kg IM.
Hepatitis A exposure: Administer ISG 0.02 ml/kg IM for exposure through close personal contact, employee at day care center, or contaminated food within 2 wks.

Tetanus Immunization

Previous tetanus immunizations	Tetanus prone wound	Non tetanus prone wound
Uncertain or <3	DT[1], TIG[2]	dT[1]
3 or more	dT if >5y since last dose	dT if >10y since last dose

[1]dT if ≥7 yo and DT if <7 yo (D contains 2X the diphtheria dose of d). [2]Tetanus immune globulin
Dose of tetanus immune globulin (TIG): Age ≥ 7 yo: 250 units IM at site other than for dT. Age <7 yo: 4 units/kg, although 250 units IM may be appropriate since the same amount of toxin will be produced in the child's body regardless of size.

Postexposure Rabies Prophylaxis

Rabies prophylaxis is only indicated if there is a bite or other salivary exposure from a carnivore or bat in household. Do not prophylax if nonsalivary exposure or bird, reptile, or rodent. HDCV (human diploid cell vaccine) dose is 1 ml IM on days 0, 3, 7, 14, & 28. Administer in thigh of young child and deltoid if older. RIG (rabies immune globulin) dose is 20 Int'l units/kg, with ½ infiltrated SC around wound and remainder in the gluteus IM. Do not give near site of the 1st HDCV injection.

		Is animal a dog or cat?	
		YES	NO, other
Was Animal captured?	NO, escaped	Give RIG & HDCV only if rabies risk for given species in locale.	Treat with RIG and full course of HDCV.
	YES, captured	Observe animal for 10 d. If abnormal behavior, sacrifice + treat patient with RIG & HDCV. Stop treatment if animal pathology negative for rabies.	Sacrifice animal + begin RIG and HDCV. Discontinue treatment if pathology negative for rabies.

Most Frequent Bacterial Pathogens and Initial Empiric Antibiotic Choice

Infection	Age	Most common etiology	Empiric antibiotics	Initial dose (maximum)
Cellulitis, face	any	S aureus, strep A, Spneumo, Hflu	cefotaxime (Claforan)	50 mg/kg IV up to 2g
Cellulitis, nonfacial	any	S aureus, strep A	cefazolin (Ancef) or nafcillin (Unipen) OR dicloxacillin, E-mycin, cephalexin	50 mg/kg IV up to 2g (see page62 for oral dosing)
Cellulitis, cat or dog bite	any	pasteurella multocida, S aureus, GNR, anaerobes	ampicillin/sulbactam (Unasyn) or penicillin G AND either (cefazolin (Ancef) or nafcillin (Unipen) OR amox-clav or (pen VK+dicloxacillin)	50-75 mg/kg IV up to 3 g 15,000-20,000 units/kg IV; 50 mg/kg IV up to 2g; (see page 62 for oral dosing)
Meningitis	0-2m	strep B, GNR, listeria, H flu type b	ampicillin AND (1) cefotaxime (Claforan) or (2) gentamicin	50-100 mg/kg IV up to 2g; 50 mg/kg IV up to 2g 2.5 mg/kg IV
	>2m	S pneumo, N meningitidis, H flu type b	cefotaxime (Claforan) or ceftriaxone (Rocephin) AND vancomycin	50 mg/kg IV up to 2g 100 mg/kg IV up to 4g 15 mg/kg IV up to 500 mg
Neutropenic fever	Any	S aureus, GNR, pseudomonas, viral, fungi, parasitic	ceftazidime(Fortaz) OR ticarcillin/clavulanate(Timentin) AND gentamicin or tobramycin ADD vancomycin if central line	50 mg/kg IV up to 2g; 50-75 mg/kg IV up to 3 g; 1-2 mg/kg IV 10 mg/kg up to 500 mg
Omphalitis	0-2m	strep A, S aureus	cefazolin (Ancef) or nafcillin (Unipen) AND gentamicin	50 mg/kg IV up to 2g; 2.5 mg/kg IV
Osteomyelitis	0-2m	S aureus, strep B, gonococcus, GNR	cefazolin (Ancef) or nafcillin (Unipen) AND gentamicin AND ampicillin	50 mg/kg IV up to 2g; 2.5 mg/kg IV; 50-100 mg/kg IV up to 2g
	>2m	S aureus, H flu, strep A	cefuroxime (Zinacef) and/or (cefazolin or nafcillin)	25-35 mg/kg IV up to 1.5g; 50 mg/kg IV up to 2g
Otitis media or sinusitis	0-1m	S pneumo, H flu, GNR	see meningitis above	see meningitis above
	>1m	S pneumo, H flu-non b, Moraxella	Amoxil, Augmentin, macrolide¹, Septra	or Rocephin 50mg/kg IM (2g)

Most Frequent Bacterial Pathogens and Initial Empiric Antibiotic Choice, continued

Infection	Age	Most common etiology	Empiric antibiotics	First dose (maximum dose)
Pharyngitis	any	strep A	benzathine penicillin or penicillin VK or macrolide[1]	30,000 units/kg IM up to 2.4 million units
	esp >2y			
Pneumonia	0-4w	Group B strep, GNR	see meningitis above	see meningitis above
	4w-3m	S pneumo, H flu, S aureus, chlamydia	cefuroxime (Zinacef) OR cefotaxime or ceftriaxone[2]	25-35 mg/kg IV up to 1.5g; 50 mg/kg IV up to 2g
	3m-3y	S pneumo, H flu	cefuroxime OR cefotaxime or ceftriaxone, OR macrolide[1] amoxicillin, amox-clav, erytho-sulfa, trimethoprim-sulfa	25-35 mg/kg IV up to 1.5g; 50 mg/kg IV up to 2g (see page XX for oral dose)
	>3y	S pneumo, mycoplasma	cefotaxime or ceftriaxone[2] OR macrolide[1] amoxicillin-clav	50 mg/kg IV up to 2g (see page 54 for oral dosing)
Septic arthritis	0-2m	Group B strep, S aureus	cefazolin or nafcillin AND gentamicin	50 mg/kg IV up to 2g; 2.5 mg/kg IV
(may need joint irrigation)	3m-3y	H flu, S aureus	cefazolin or nafcillin	50 mg/kg IV up to 2g;
	> 3 y	S aureus, strep A,S pneumo, H flu, gonococcus (esp. > 12 y)	AND cefotaxime or ceftriaxone	50 mg/kg IV up to 2g
Sepsis	-	see meningitis	see meningitis	see meningitis above
Urinary tract	0-2 mo	E coli, GNR, enterococcus, staph	ampicillin AND gentamicin	50 mg/kg IV up to 2 g 2.5 mg/kg IV
	> 2 mo	E coli, GNR, enterococcus, staph	ceftriaxone or cefotaxime	50 mg/kg IV up to 2 g

Tailor treatment accordingly if other pathogens, antibiotic resistance, or allergy. Changes are indicated if immunosuppression, underlying disease, or specific bacterial pathogen known. Consult recent literature, standard textbooks, and specialists when uncertain about optimal therapy. GNR = gram negative rods, S pneumo - *Streptococcus pneumoniae*, S aureus - *Staphylococcus aureus*, strep - streptococcus.
[1]macrolides - azithromycin (*Zithromax*), clarithromycin (*Biaxin*), erythromycin. [2]Add macrolide if chlamydia or mycoplasma suspected.

Common Oral Antimicrobial Doses and Mixtures

Antimicrobial	Formulations	Dose (Frequency) [1]
amoxicillin (*Amoxil*)	Susp: 125, 250 mg/5ml Caps: 125, 250 mg	30-50 mg/kg/day (tid) Max dose 500 mg
amoxicillin/clavulanate (*Augmentin*)	Susp: 200 & 400 mg/5ml Tabs: 250, 500 mg	45 mg/kg/day (bid) Max dose 500 mg
ampicillin (*Polycillin*)	Susp: 125, 250 mg/5ml Caps: 250, 500 mg	50-100 mg/kg/day (qid) Max dose 500 mg
azithromycin[2] (*Zithromax*)	Susp: 100, 200, 1000 mg/5ml Caps: 250 mg, 1000 mg	10 mg/kg qd on 1st day, then 5 mg/kg qd x 4d pharyngitis 12mg/kg/d X5d Max dose 500 mg
cefaclor (*Ceclor*) 2nd generation	Susp: 125, 250 mg/5ml Caps: 250, 500 mg	20-40 mg/kg/day (tid) Max dose 500 mg
cefadroxil (*Duricef*) 1st generation	Susp: 125,250,500 mg/5ml Cap: 500, Tab: 1000 mg	30 mg/kg/day (bid) Max dose 1000 mg
cefixime (*Suprax*) 3rd generation	Syrup: 100 mg/5ml Tabs: 200, 400 mg	8 mg/kg/day (qd/bid) Max dose 400 mg
cefpodoxime (*Vantin*) 3rd generation	Susp: 50, 100 mg/5ml Tabs: 100, 200 mg	10 mg/kg/day (bid) Max dose 400 mg
cefprozil (*Cefzil*) 3rd generation	Susp: 125, 250 mg/5ml Tabs: 250 mg/5ml	15 mg/kg/day (bid) Max dose 500 mg
ceftibuten (*Cedax*) 3rd generation	Susp: 90, 180 mg/5ml Caps: 400 mg	9 mg/dg/day (qd) Max dose 400 mg
cefuroxime (*Ceftin*) 2nd generation	Susp: 125 mg/5ml Tabs: 125, 250, 500 mg	15-30 mg/kg/day (bid) Max dose 500 mg
cephalexin (*Keflex*) 1st generation	Susp: 125, 250 mg/5ml Caps: 250, 500 mg	25-50 mg/kg/day (qid) Max dose 500 mg
clarithromycin (*Biaxin*)	Susp: 125, 250 mg/5 ml Tabs: 250, 500 mg	15 mg/kg/day (bid) Max dose 500 mg
clindamycin (*Cleocin*)	Solution: 75 mg/5ml Cap: 75,150 mg	10-25 mg/kg/day (tid/bid) Max dose 600 mg
dicloxacillin (*Dynapen*)	Susp: 62.5 mg/5ml Caps: 125, 250, 500	25-100 mg/kg/day (qid) Max dose 500 mg
erythromycin (*ERYC, EES, E-mycin*)	Susp: 200, 400 mg/5ml Tab: 200(chew),250,400,500	20-50 mg/kg/day (qid) Max dose 500 mg
erythromycin/sulfisox- azole (*Pediazole*)	Susp: 200 mg EM & 600 mg SS per 5ml	50 mg EM/kg/day (qid) Max EM dose 500 mg

[1]Max Dose = Maximum individual oral dose   [2]20mg/kg X 1 dose required for Chlamydia

Common Oral Antimicrobial Doses and Mixtures

Antimicrobial	Formulations	Dose (Frequency)
fluconazole (*Diflucan*)	Susp: 10, 40 mg/ml Tabs: 50, 100, 200 mg	3-6 mg/kg/day (qd) Max dose 200 mg
furazolidone (*Furoxone*)	Susp: 50 mg/5ml Tabs: 100 mg	6 mg/kg/d X 10 days Max dose 400 mg/d
griseofulvin (*Grifulvin V*)	Susp: 125 mg/5ml Caps: 125, 250 mg Tabs: 125, 250, 500 mg Max dose 1000 mg	15-20 mg/kg/day (qd) <u>tinea corporis</u> X 2 wk <u>tinea pedis/manus</u> X 4 wk <u>tinea capitis</u> X 6 weeks
loracarbef (*Lorabid*) 2nd generation	Susp: 100, 200 mg/5ml Caps: 200 mg	15-30 mg/kg/day (bid) Max dose 400 mg
mebendazole (*Vermox*)	Tabs: 100 mg chewable	<u>pinworms:</u> 100 mg X1, repeat in 2 weeks
metronidazole (*Flagyl*)	Tabs: 250, 500 mg	<u>Giardia:</u>15 mg/kg/day (tid) X 7 days
nitrofurantoin (*Macrodantin*)	Susp: 25 mg/5ml, Tab: 50,100 mg Caps: 25, 50, 100 mg	5-7 mg/kg/day (qid) Max dose 100 mg
nystatin (*Mycostatin*)	Susp: 100,000 units/ml Tabs: 500,000 units Max dose 500,000 units	<u>Neo:</u> 1ml q cheek (qid) until clear X 48 hours <u>Children:</u> 500,000 units qid until clear X 48 hrs
penicillin (*Pen-Vee K*)	Susp: 125, 250 Tab: 125, 250, 500 mg	25-50 mg/kg/day (qid) Max dose 500 mg
sulfisoxazole (*Gantrisin*)	Susp: 500 mg/5ml Tab: 500 mg	120-150 mg/kg/day (qid) Max dose 1000 mg
trimethoprim / sulfa- methoxazole (*Bactrim, Septra*)	Susp: 40 mg TMP & 200 mg SMX per 5ml Tabs: 80/400, 160/800	6-12 mg TMP & 30-60 mg SMX per kg/day (bid) Max dose 160 TMP[1]
vancomycin (*Vancocin*)	Caps: 125, 250	40 mg/kg/d X 7 d Max dose 2000 mg/d

[1]*Higher doses needed for severe UTI, shigella, and pneumocystis infections*

Recommended Antibiotic Therapy for Infectious Diarrhea

Organism	Scenario	Antimicrobial Agent (oral dose unless otherwise stated)
Aeromonas h.		TMP[1] 6-12 mg/kg/d + SMX[1] 30-60 mg/kg/d X 5 d
Campylobacter	may not need	Erythromycin 40 mg/kg/d X 7 d
Clostridia dificil	mild	None
	severe	Metronidazole 30 mg/kg/d X 7 d (max 750 mg/d) or Vancomycin 20 mg/kg/d X 7 d (max 300 mg/d)
E. coli	enterotoxin	None
	invasive	TMP[1] 6-12 mg/kg/d + SMX[1] 30-60 mg/kg/d X 5 d
Giardia		Furazolidone 6 mg/kg/d X 10 d Or metronidazole 15 mg/kg/d X 10 days (max 750 mg/d)
Salmonella	uncomplicated	None
	complicated[2]	Ampicillin 100 mg/kg/d IV X 10 d Or TMP[1] 6-12 mg/kg/d + SMX[1] 30-60 mg/kg/d X 10 d
Shigella		TMP[1] 6-12 mg/kg/d + SMX[1] 30-60 mg/kg/d X 5 d Or Ampicillin 100 mg/kg/d X 5 d
Vibrio cholera		TMP[1] 6-12 mg/kg/d + SMX[1] 30-60 mg/kg/d X 3 d
Yersinia		TMP[1] 6-12 mg/kg/d + SMX[1] 30-60 mg/kg/d X 5 d

[1] TMX - trimethoprim, SMX - sulfamethoxazole; TMP/SMX - *Septra*

[2] complicated - infants < 3-6 months old, disseminated, bacteremia,
   immunocompromised, enteric fever   *Emerg Med Clin North Am* 1995; 436.

Topical Ectoparasiticides

lindane (*Kwell, Scabene*)	cream1% (10mg/g;60g) lotion 1% (10mg/ml; 30,60,480ml) DO NOT USE if < 2 yo	P. capitis: Massage into hair, leave on X 10 min, rinse & dry. Comb nits. Scabies: Apply from chin to toes. Wash off in 6 h. Repeat in 1 wk.
Permethrin (*Nix, Elimite*) More effective than lindane vs. Scabies	cream5% (60 g: *Elimite*) liquid 1% (60 ml: *Nix*) DO NOT USE if <2 MONTHS OLD	P. capitis: Wash hair, then saturate hair, leave on 10 min, then rinse and comb out nits and lice. Scabies: Apply cream to entire body, wash off in 8-12 h. Repeat in 1 wk.

Postexposure Prophylaxis to Select Infectious Agents

Exposure	Who should receive prophylaxis	Management
Haemophilus influenzae type b	• All house contacts, if a child < 4 years old lives at home • Day care center contact < 2 years • Day care staff/attendees if ≥ 2 cases occurred within 6 months	Rifampin 20 mg/kg/qd X 4 Max dose 600 mg Decrease to 10 mg/kg if < 1 month old
Neisseria meningitidis	• All household, day care, or nursery contacts within 24h of index case • Older children and adults if they kissed, shared food, or drank from same container with index case • Med personnel exposed to secretion	Rifampin 5 mg/kg q12h X 4 Max dose 600 mg May substitute sulfisoxazole if organism is sensitive to sulfa or ciprofloxacin 500 mg single dose in adults.
Measles	• All persons *susceptible* to measles > 12 months old who are exposed • *Susceptible* = all persons unless they have a documented measles case, were born before 1957, lab evidence of immunity, or completed appropriate live-virus vaccination. **DO NOT** give live attenuated vaccine if Neomycin allergy, TB, immuno-suppressed, chronic steroid use, heme-cancer, pregnancy or ≤ 3 months from blood, plasma or Immunoglobulin use.	Live measles vaccine if ≤ 72 h of exposure prevents disease. Use monovalent vaccine if 6-12 months old. Use *Immune globulin* (IG) for immunosuppressed or pregnant: (1) 0.25 ml/kg (max 15 ml) IM within 6 days exposure. (2) Double dose (max 15 ml) for immunocompromised. (3) Give measles vaccine no sooner than 5 months after IG.
Rubella	Only prophylax pregnant > 13 weeks	Immune globulinIG 0.55 ml/kg IM
Varicella	• Significant exposure to immuno-compromised children (also HIV+) without prior chicken pox • Susceptible pregnant women • newborn with mom's chicken pox on-set ≤ 5d pre to 2days post delivery • Hospitalized premature infants ≥ 28 weeks whose mom has no history of chicken pox, is seronegative or new-born< 28 weeks regardless of mom's history who is exposed to varicella	Varicella immune globulin (VZIG) should be administered within 96 hours of exposure. *Newborn:* VZIG 125 U IM. *Older:* 125 U/10 kg (max 625 U)
AAP Committee on Infectious Disease. 1997	All children > 12 years, or with chronic cutaneous or pulmonary disorders, or on chronic salicylate therapy Pregnancy is not an indication (effective within 24-48 h of exposure)	Acyclovir 20 mg/kg PO qid X 5d (maximum dose 800 mg) Tabs: 200, 400, 800 Susp: 200 mg/5 ml (Zovirax)

Clinical Scoring for Group A Streptococcal Pharyngitis

Fever > 38.3C (101F)	Each of 6 features	Total	PPV[1]
Age 5-15 years	is worth one point	1	0%
Nov-May presentation	(mnemonic = FANCUP)	2 or 3	20%
Cervical adenopathy		4	42%
URI absent (i.e., cough, rhinorrhea, congestion)		5	63%
Pharyngitis (i.e., tonsillar erythema, hypertrophy, or exudate)		6	75%

[1]PPV=Positive predictive value for Group A streptococcus   *Pediatr Emerg Care 1998; 14: 109.*

Yale Observation Scale

Observation item	Normal (score 1 point)	Moderate impairment (score 3 points)	Severe impairment (score 5 points)
Quality of cry	strong or none	whimper or sob	weak, moaning, high-pitched, hardly responds
Reaction to parents	cries briefly, no crying, content	cries off and on	persistent cry with little response
State variation	awake, or if asleep wakens quickly	eyes close briefly, awake or wakens with prolonged stimulation	no arousal, falls asleep
Color	pink	pale extremities, acrocyanosis	pale, cyanotic, mottled, or ashen
Hydration	Normal skin eyes, mouth	Normal skin and eyes, mouth slightly dry	Skin doughy/tented, dry mouth, sunken eyes
Response overtures	alert or smiles (consistently)	alert or brief smile	no smile, anxious, dull no alerting to overtures

Rates of Serious Illness & Bacteremia in Febrile Children 3-36 months old

Serious illness rate		Bacteremia rate if temp ≥ 39ºC	
Yale < 10	2.7%	Yale = 6	2.5%
Yale 11-15	26%	Yale ≥ 8	4.7%
Yale > 16	92.3%	Yale ≥ 10	5.7%

McCarthy: Pediatrics 1982;70:802   Teach, Fleisher: J Pediatrics 1995; 877

Clinical Features in Bacterial Meningitis

History[1]	Frequency	Exam[1]	Frequency	Nuchal rigidity[2]	
History fever	• 95%	Temp ≥38.3C	• 59-77%	Age	Frequency
Lethargy or Irritability	• 87-95%	Altered LOC	• 53-78%	0-6 months	27%
		ENT infection	• 22-44%	7-12 months	71%
Vomiting	• 54-71%	Focal deficit	• 5-6%	13-18 months	87%
URI	• 46-55%			> 18 months	95%

[1]*Ann Emerg Med 1992;21:146.*   [2]*Ann Emerg Med 1992;21:911.*

Rochester Criteria for Febrile Infants (28-90 days)

1. No skeletal, soft tissue, or ear infection	5. UA <10 WBC's/HPF
2. WBC 5,000-15,000, bands <1,500	6. If diarrhea, stool <5 WBC's/HPF
3. Born full term	7. Normal CSF
4. No prior hospitalizations, antibiotics, hyperbilirubinemia, or underlying illness.	

Serious bacterial infection occur in 7-9% of well-appearing infants 28-90 days old.
If *all* of the above Rochester criteria are present, the incidence is <1%.

J Pediatr 1985;107:855, Pediatr Infect Dis J 1992;11:257

Occult Bacteremia

Temp (°C)	Temp (°F)	Incidence	
< 39.4	< 102.9	1.6%	Incidence of + blood cultures in
39.5-39.9	103-103.8	2.1%	nontoxic febrile children 3-36
40-41	104-105.8	3.5%	months of age with no source
> 41	> 105.8	9.3%	*Harper Pediatr Ann 1993; 22: 484*

Temp. conversion °C = (°F−32)(5/9)

Management of Child with Fever and No Source (*Pediatrics* 1993; 92: 1)

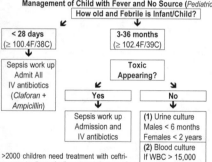

How old and Febrile is Infant/Child?

< 28 days (≥ 100.4F/38C)
→ Sepsis work up Admit All IV antibiotics (*Claforan + Ampicillin*)

3-36 months (≥ 102.4F/39C)
→ Toxic Appearing?

- **Yes** → Sepsis work up Admission and IV antibiotics
- **No** →
  (1) Urine culture Males < 6 months Females < 2 years
  (2) Blood culture If WBC > 15,000 or all > 39C
  (3) Stool culture If stool has blood or ≥ 5 WBC/hpf
  (4) CXR if focal exam abnormality or breathing fast
  (5) Empiric IM ceftriaxone 50mg/kg in all or only if ↑WBC

28-90 days (≥ 100.4F/38C)
→ If Toxic admit
→ If non-toxic assess for Rochester criteria (RC) above
→ Discharge after ceftriaxone IM if normal RC Otherwise Admit
→ Follow up all in 24-48 h

>2000 children need treatment with ceftriaxone to theoretically prevent 1 case of meningitis (causing >400 side effects) & >650 to prevent 1 serious infection For this reason, some experts only treat empirically if (1) temperature ≥ 40-41C, (2) Yale score > 6 (3) poor follow-up, (4) non-Hib immunization or (5) no minor source of infection already requiring oral antibiotics.
Pediatrics 1997;99:438;
Acad Emerg Med 1998; 5:599

Urinary Tract Infections (UTI)

	Age	UTI Risk[1]
Organisms in neonates: E coli 74%, klebsiella 7%, pseudomonas 7%, proteus 4%. In older infants/children: E coli is most common. Proteus and klebsiella occur in hospitalized, recurrent UTI, and males.	0-2 months	7.5%
	2-24 months	4.1%
	2-5 years	1.7%

[1]If fever present, regardless of symptoms

Risk factors and Symptoms of UTI in Febrile Infants and Children < 3 years old	Most Common UTI Symptoms		Risk of UTI if feature present	
	irritability	80%	female > 39 C	8.8%
	poor feeding	65%	fever without source	7.5%
	vomiting/diarrhea	30-40%	fever + otitis media	3.5%
	URI symptoms	10-20%	fever + major source	1.5%

Symptoms are poor at discriminating between fever due to UTI or other source < 3 yr.

Schlager *Pediatr Ann* 1993; 505. Hoberman *J Pediatr* 1993; 123: 17

Diagnosis: 93% of positive cultures from "bag" urines are contaminants. Nitrate dipstick + indicates E coli, proteus, klebsiella, enterobacter, salmonella; (not S. saprophyticus, pseudomonas, enterococcus). A UA is insensitive in diagnosing UTI; culture all < 3-5 yr.

Predictive Value of Urinalysis in Detecting UTI

Urinalysis feature	Sensitivity	Negative predictive value
Any WBC/high power field (hpf)	77%	97%
≥ 5 WBC/hpf	54%	97%
Any bacteria	86%	99%
+ leuk esterase,nitrate,or ≥ 5WBC/hpf	75-85%	85-97%
Positive gram stain for bacteria	94-99%	99%

Antibiotic Choices for Urinary Tract Infection

- Admit if < 3 months old, obstruction, high grade reflux, dehydration, vomiting, toxicity.
- Gentamicin 5 mg/kg/d IV divided q 12h + Ampicillin 100 mg/kg/d IV divided q 12h (esp. if gram positive bacteria on gram stain) **OR**
- Ceftriaxone 75/mg/kg/d IV divided q 12-24 h (do not use in neonates) **OR**
- Cefotaxime 150 mg/kg/d IV divided q 6-8 h.
- Oral therapy: Antibiotic choices include *Septra, Suprax, Augmentin, Keflex.* Treat for 14 days if upper tract, and 5-7 days if lower tract infection. See pages 62,63 for dose.

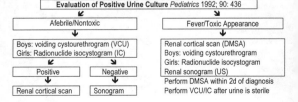

Evaluation of Positive Urine Culture *Pediatrics* 1992; 90: 436

Afebrile/Nontoxic	Fever/Toxic Appearance
Boys: voiding cystourethrogram (VCU) Girls: Radionuclide isocystogram (IC)	Renal cortical scan (DMSA) Boys: voiding cystourethrogram Girls: Radionuclide isocystogram Renal sonogram (US)

Afebrile/Nontoxic branch:
- Positive → Renal cortical scan
- Negative → Sonogram

Fever/Toxic Appearance:
Perform DMSA within 2d of diagnosis
Perform VCU/IC after urine is sterile

Kawasaki's Disease

Overview: Kawasaki's diseases is an acute vasculitis of unknown origin. Kawasaki's leads to cardiac complications in 25% of cases, and is the #1 acquired heart disease in children. The earliest sign is high fever (≥ 40°C) for up to 10 days. Small and medium arteries are affected throughout the body, with infiltration & destruction of the intima and media by macrophages, lymphocytes, and mast cells.	Phases of Kawasaki's Disease
	• *Acute phase* (0-2 weeks from onset) Sudden fever, rash, conjunctivitis, lymphadenopathy, mucosal changes, and/or myocarditis
	• *Subacute phase* (2-8 weeks) Arthritis, epidermal desquamation (beginning periungually), possibility of cardiac thrombi/aneurysm forming
	• *Convalescent phase* (up to 2 years) - Risk of coronary aneurysm formation

Diagnostic Criteria[1]

Fever lasting at least 5 days without other source, and at least 4 of the following:

- Bilateral conjunctival injection (painless, and without exudate)
- Mucous membrane changes (e.g., injected pharynx, strawberry tongue, or redness, fissuring, and crusting of lips)
- Edema or erythema of palms or soles (desquamation in convalescent phase)
- Rash (polymorphous and truncal)
- Cervical adenopathy, with at least one node > 1.5 cm

[1]Other *nondiagnostic* features: sleep disturbances (90%), urethritis and sterile pyuria (75%), uveitis/iritis (80%) arthralgias/arthritis (~30%), or hemolytic uremic syndrome (rare)

Diagnostic Tests

- Platelet count > 1 million, during (subacute) thrombosis stage, normal acutely
- Leukocytosis, with left shift, mild hemolytic anemia, CRP and ESR elevation
- Urine - Moderate pyuria, occasional bilirubinuria due to gallbladder hydrops
- CXR – Cardiomegaly in up to 30%
- EKG – 1st week: low voltage, ST depression, 2nd-3rd week: PR and QT prolongation, ST elevation

Evaluation and treatment

- Gamma globulin: Administer 2 grams/kg IV over 8-12 h as a single infusion.
- Aspirin: 80-100 mg/kg/day PO divided qid until 14th day of illness, then 3-5 mg/kg PO qd until 6-8 weeks after onset. If coronary artery aneurysm is evident on echocardiogram, continuation of ASA beyond 8 weeks may be indicated.
- Obtain echocardiogram on presentation. Repeat 14, 21 and 60 days after onset.

Renal Disorders

<u>Urinalysis</u>: False + dipstick for blood occur with UTI's, betadine, ascorbic acid. RBC casts or dysmorphic RBC's suggest glomerular disease. Infants < 3 months old cannot concentrate urine well, therefore, specific gravity is unreliable at this age.

Differential Diagnosis of Hematuria

- *Extrarenal disorders*: coagulation disorders, salicylates, sickle cell disease/trait
- *Renal extraglomerular*: hemorrhagic cystitis, trauma, nephrolithiasis, familial hypercalciuria, nephritis, hydronephrosis, polycystic kidneys, renal vein thrombosis, papillary necrosis, hemangiomas, tumor (e.g., Wilm's), foreign body, posterior urethral valves, ureteropelvic junction obstruction, renal tuberculosis.
- *Renal glomerular*: glomerulonephritis, IgA nephropathy, Alport's syndrome, exercise, familial benign hematuria, focal glomerulosclerosis.
- *Systemic*: allergy, hepatitis B antigenemia, endocarditis, cardiac shunt or valve, Henoch-Schonlein purpura, hemolytic uremic syndrome, polyarteritis.

Causes of Red Urine

Hematuria, alcaptonuria, bilirubinemia, phenazopyridine, phenothiazines, *Motrin*, L-dopa, phenolphthalein, methyldopa, adriamycin, deferoxamine, *Dilantin*, quinine, sulfa, chloroform, naphthalene, oxalic acid, anilines, food color, beets, blueberries, rhubarb, fava beans, hemoglobinuria or myoglobinuria (Heme + dipstick with no RBC's), porphyrins, red diaper syndrome (*serratia*), tyrosinosis.

Normal Bladder Volume and Normal Plasma Creatinine (PCr)

Bladder volume Estimate	• < 1 year old: weight (kg) X 10 ml • > 1 year old: (age in years + 2) x 30 ml
Plasma Creatinine Estimate	• *Males*: PCr (mg/dl) = 0.35 + (0.025 x age in years) • *Females*: PCr (mg/dl) = 0.35 + (0.018 x age in years)

Differentiating Between Causes of Renal Failure

Test	Pre-renal	Renal	Post-renal
Urine sodium	< 20	> 40	> 40
Fractional excretion of sodium[1]	< 1	> 2	> 2
Renal failure index[2]	< 1	> 2	> 2
Urine osmolality	> 500	< 300	< 400
Urine/serum creatinine ratio	> 40	< 20	< 20
Serum BUN/creatinine ratio	> 20	< 10-20	< 10-20
Renal size by ultrasound	normal	normal	normal or ↑
Radionuclide renal scan	↓uptake ↓excretion	uptake OK ↓excretion	uptake OK ↓excretion

[1] FE_{Na} = 100 x (urine Na$^+$/plasma Na$^+$) / (urine creatinine/plasma creatinine)
  Normal FE_{Na} is 1-2%, except under 2 months when FE_{Na} up may be to 5%.
[2] RFI = (urine Na$^+$) / (urine creatinine / serum creatinine)

Neurology

Assessment of Coma and Altered Level of Consciousness

Trauma or tumor Infection/Intussusception Poisons Sepsis, Seizure, Shock	Abuse or alcohol Encephalopathy/Endocrine Insulin/hypoglycemia or metabolic error Opiates Uremia	*Differential Diagnosis of Coma & ALOC* mnemonic **TIPS-AEIOU**

	Infant	Child	Adolescent

**Common Causes
of Altered Mental
Status by Age**
	Infection
	Metabolic (inborn or
	    acquired disorder)
	Abuse
		Ingestion
		Infection
		Intussusception
		Seizure/abuse
			Ingestion
			Trauma
			Poison (drug,
			    alcohol use)

Treatment of Infant/Child with an Altered Mental Status

- Assess airway and breathing (immobilizing cervical spine if possible trauma).
- Consider endotracheal intubation if poor or labored respiratory effort, diminished airway reflexes, suspicion of elevated ICP, or severe hypoxemia.
- Assess pulse oximetry and administer 100% oxygen.
- Obtain rapid glucose measurement or administer glucose (dosage, page 3).
- Administer naloxone 0.1 mg/kg.
- Measure child's length to facilitate dosing and sizing of equipment (see page 3).
- Complete vital signs: temp, respirations, pulse, & BP. Perform complete exam.
- Direct further evaluation based on above measures, and history + examination.

Normal Neonatal/Infant Reflexes Appearance/Disappearance

Reflex (description)	Appears	Disappears
Moro - lift head 30° and let fall to neutral. A positive test = arm extension and abduction, then arm adduction	Birth	1-3 months
Palmar grasp - object in hand causes flexion/grasping	Birth	4 months
Root response - stroking cheek causes mouth to turn in direction of stimulus	Birth	3-4 months
Tonic neck - turn head to side while child is supine, with ipsilateral arm & leg extending and opposite arm/leg flexing. Normal infant tries to break reflex position.	Birth	5-6 months
+ *Babinski* - stroking lateral border of sole, to big toe. Pos. reflex causes big toe dorsiflexion, + fanning of other toes.	Birth	1-2 years

Most Common Etiologies	Viral illness	39%	Strep throat	5%
of Headache in Children	Sinusitis	16%	Tension	5%
Presenting to a Pediatric	Migraine	16%	Other disease	8%
Emergency Department	Post-trauma	7%	Serious CNS	
Pediatr Emerg Care 1997;13:1.	Viral meningitis	5%	disorders[1]	7%

[1] includes 5% viral meningitis, and < 0.3% each of bleed, tumor, hydrocephalus

---

Seizures and Status Epilepticus

Most Common Seizure Etiology by Age

Day 1	
Hypoxia (perinatal-intrauterine)	Hyopglycemia, Hyperglycemia
Birth trauma (subarachnoid, subdural)	Infection (group B streptococcus, E. coli)
Drugs (e.g. cocaine)	Pyridoxine deficiency

Days 2 - 3	
Hypoxia	Developmental malformations
Infection	Intracranial hemorrhage
Drug withdrawal (esp. narcotics)	Inborn errors of metabolism (days 4-14)
Hypoglycemia, Hypocalcemia (day 3-14)	Hyponatremia, Hypernatremia

Days 4 - 28	
Infection	Developmental malformations
Hypocalcemia (esp. days 3-14)	Drug withdrawal (esp. narcotics)
Hyperphosphatemia	Inborn errors of metabolism (days 4-14)
Hyponatremia	aminoaciduria, organic aciduria, urea cycle

Months 1-6 (same as month 1)	

Year 0.5 - 3	
Febrile seizures, Birth injury	Trauma, metabolic disorder
Infection, or Toxin	Cerebral degeneration

> 3 Years	
Idiopathic	Trauma
Infection	Cerebral degeneration

Seizure Mimics

Infant	Child[1]	Adolescent[1]
jitteriness (withdrawal), tremor	breath holding	vagal syncope, orthostasis
apnea (> 20 sec with cyanosis)	micturition,cough syncope	migraine
micturitional shivering	night tremor, terror	hyperventilation
dysrhythmia	migraine	pseudoseizures
Sandifer syndrome (GE reflux)	tics	hysteria

[1]in general patients have precipitant, premonitory symptoms, and are not post-ictal

Management of Status Epilepticus

- Protect airway, administer O_2, start IV, attach cardiac monitor and pulse oximeter, and have intubation equipment prepared.
- Perform stat bedside glucose test and send electrolytes and drug levels.
- Administer IV glucose if hypoglycemia (10 ml/kg of $D_{10}W$ if a neonate, 4 ml/kg of $D_{25}W$ if <2 yo, 2 ml/kg of $D_{50}W$ if >2 yo), and thiamine 100 mg if malnourished.
- Intravenous drug therapy as per table. If the first drug is unsuccessful, try another agent. If this is unsuccessful, consider general anesthesia.
- Treat fever and correct sodium, calcium, or magnesium abnormalities.

Intravenous Drug Therapy for Status Epilepticus (A-D preferred order)

	Drug	Dose & route	Maximum rate	Special features
A	lorazepam	0.05-0.15 mg/kg IV	<0.5-1 mg/min	may repeat q5 min x2
	or diazepam	0.2-0.3 mg/kg IV	<1.0 mg/min	may repeat q5 min x2
	or diazepam	0.5 mg/kg PR	--	may repeat ½ dose x1
B	fosphenytoinPE[1]	15-18 mg/kg IV	< 2 mg/kg/min	monitor closely
	or phenytoin	15-18 mg/kg IV	< 0.5 mg/kg/min	monitor closely
C	phenobarbital	15-30 mg/kg IV	< 1.0 mg/kg/min	monitor closely
D	pentobarbital	2-10 mg/kg (IV load)	slow IV	intubation required;
	(coma)	0.5-3.0 mg/kg/h	< 1 mg/kg min	vasopressors prn

[1] PE – phenytoin equivalents

Oral Anticonvulsants

Drug	Indications	Oral dose[1]	IV load (mg/kg)	Level[2] (µg/ml)	Half-life (h)
carbamazepine (*Tegretol*):tabs 100, 200 mg; susp: 100mg/5ml	grand mal, partial, psychomotor	15-30	-	4-14	12
clonazepam (*Klonopin*), tabs 0.5, 1, 2 mg	myoclonic, atonic	0.01-0.02	-	0.013-0.072	18-50
ethosuximide (*Zarontin*), syrup 250 mg/5ml, cap 250 mg	petit mal	20-30	-	40-100	30
phenobarbital, elixir 20 mg/5ml, tabs 15,30,60,90,100 mg	grand mal	3-5	15-20[3]	10-35	48-72
phenytoin (*Dilantin*), susp 30 & 125 mg/5ml, tab 30,50,100 mg	grand mal, partial, psychomotor	5-10	15-20[4]	10-20	6-30
primidone (*Mysoline*), susp 250 mg/5ml, tab 50,250 mg	grand mal, partial, psychomotor	10-25	6-12	5-12	48-72
valproate (*Depakene*), syrup 250 mg/5ml, cap 250 mg	petit or grand mal, myoclonic, atonic	15-60	-	50-100	6-16

[1]Total daily maintenance dose in mg/kg. [2]Therapeutic. [3]No faster than 1 mg/kg/min. [4]No faster than 0.5 mg/kg/min.

Acute Weakness

Upper motor neuron (UMN) lesions cause damage to the cortex (e.g., stroke), brain stem, or spinal cord. Lower motor neuron (LMN) lesions damage the anterior horn cells (e.g., poliomyelitis), the neuromuscular junction (e.g., myasthenia gravis, botulism toxin) or muscle (e.g., muscular dystrophies).

	Category	_UMN disease_	_LMN disease_
Differentiation of	Muscular deficit	Muscle groups	Individual muscles
upper motor neuron	Reflexes	Increased	Decreased/absent
from lower motor	Tone	Increased	Decreased
neuron disease	Fasciculations	Absent	Present
	Atrophy	Absent/minimal	Present

Ataxia

Ataxia is the incoordination of movement with normal strength. Disorders of the cerebellar hemispheres cause ipsilateral limb ataxia, while disorders of the vermis cause truncal ataxia. Other causes of acute ataxia include cerebral cortex disorders (frontal ataxia), peripheral sensory nerve and spinal cord disorders (sensory ataxia), labyrinth disorders (vestibular ataxia), metabolic, and toxin-induced ataxia.

Specific diseases causing ataxia

- Acute cerebellar ataxia - the most common cause of acute ataxia in children. This is a post-viral autoimmune ataxia typically occurring in 1-3 yr olds 2-3 weeks after varicella, influenza, or coxsackie infections. This disorder causes a sudden onset of ataxia, nystagmus in 50%, elevated CSF protein, mild CSF pleocytosis, and frequently dysarthria. Ataxia may persist for weeks to years in up to 1/3 of patients.
- Drug ingestion - Common drugs causing ataxia include phenytoin (and most anticonvulsants), alcohol, tricyclic antidepressants, hypnotics, sedatives, heavy metals (e.g., lead), insecticides and drugs of abuse (e.g., PCP).
- Neuroblastomas - Occult neuroblastomas can cause classic triad of symptoms with acute ataxia, opsoclonus (jerky, random eye movements), and myoclonus.
- Posterior fossa tumors - Direct cerebellar involvement or hydrocephalus
- Diseases causing weakness easily mistaken for ataxia including Guillain-Barre, transverse myelitis, tick paralysis, and myasthenia gravis.
- Other causes include head trauma, stroke, vasculitis, and congenital disorders.

Nutrition

Water comprises 75% of body weight in infants and 60% in adults.

Energy requirements

A child under 12 months of age requires 105-115 kcal/kg/day. Breast milk or commercially prepared infant formulas are usually the sole source of energy and nutrients in the first few months of life. Semisolid foods (e.g., cereals) are usually introduced into the diet at 4-6 months of age and soft table foods at 1 year.

Breast milk

Breast milk is preferred over formula by the American Academy of Pediatrics. Breast-fed infants have lower mortality, fewer respiratory infections, less otitis media, and less diarrhea compared with formula-fed infants. Breast-fed infants also require fewer calories than formula-fed infants. Lactose is the predominant carbohydrate in breast milk, although glucose and galactose are also found. Human milk has lower protein concentrations than cow's milk (0.9% vs. 3.4%), and is more easily digested than cow milk as the casein:whey ratio is lower (40/60 vs. 80/20). A disadvantage of breast feeding is infant jaundice due to the inhibitory effects of a progesterone metabolite on bilirubin conjugation. This physiologic jaundice generally appears after the third day of life, peaks in the first week, and is usually associated with bilirubin levels of 10-27 mg/dl (although levels >15 may be concerning, see page 46). Contraindications to breast feeding include maternal (1) eclampsia, (2) severe infection, (3) TB, (4) severe heart disease, (5) thyrotoxicosis, (6) diabetes mellitus, (6) chronic renal disease, or (7) severe puerperal depression. Mastitis is not a contraindication.

Infant formulas

Most infant formulas supply 20 calories per ounce. AAP recommends formulas with caloric distribution of 30-54% fat, 7-18% protein, and remainder from carbohydrates. If fluoridated drinking water is not available, then fluoride supplementation is recommended for all infants. Iron supplementation is recommended by the AAP after 4 months of age because of normally depleted iron stores. Most formulas contain 1 mg/L iron and fortified formulas contain 10-12 mg/L (beware of constipation).

Low birth weight infants

Preterm and low birth-weight infants require 120-180 kcal/kg/day and 3 g/kg/day of protein to maintain growth and adequate nutritional status. The composition of breast milk produced by preterm mothers is uniquely suited to preterm or low birth weight neonates, and differs substantially from that produced at term.

Weaning and mixed feeding

Beginning at 5-6 months of age, it is recommended that mothers gradually replace one breast feeding at a time with a formula feed offered by bottle or cup. Weaning is more easily accepted by an infant who has already been spoon-fed some solid foods. By 12 months of age, most infants have settled into a schedule of 3-4 meals per day. While bovine milk formulas are acceptable, regular bovine milk should not be given until after 1 year of age. Caries can occur from repetitive, prolonged (e.g., overnight) sucking of bottles before 2 years of age.

First year feeding problems

- *Constipation* is rare in breast-fed infants. Formulas high in fat and protein may promote constipation. For these infants, increasing the amount of fluid or sugar by adding one or two teaspoons of *Karo* syrup to eight ounces of water is usually helpful. In children over 4 months, add bulk such as cereal, vegetables, or fruit. Discontinue iron-fortified formula, as they exacerbate constipation.
- *Colic* is rare after 3 months of age.

Nutritional Disorders

Failure to thrive (FTT)

Inadequate growth is indicated by a weight that is $\leq$ the 3rd-5th percentile on standard growth chart or < 80-85% of the median for that child's age or height. Risk factors: young mother (<17 yo), social isolation, marital problems, and poverty.

Bovine milk allergy

The prevalence of allergy to bovine (cow's) milk has been reported at 0.3% - 7.5%. Allergy is due to sensitivity to the primary protein in bovine milk, β-lactoglobulin. Infants with milk allergy usually present during the 1st 6 weeks of life with diarrhea, mucous or bloody stools, and occasional respiratory symptoms. Treatment is aimed at eliminating bovine milk protein from the diet and substituting soy-based (e.g., *Progestimil*) or hydrolyzed casein formulas (e.g., *Nutramigen*).

Normal Feeding Amount and Timing

Age	Volume of meal (ounces)	Frequency
0 - 2 weeks	2 - 3	q 2 - 3 hours
2 - 6 weeks	3 - 4	q 3 - 4 hours
1 - 3 months	5 - 6	q 4 - 5 hours
3 - 4 months	6 - 7	q 5 - 6 hours
4 - 8 months	7 - 8	q 6 - 7 hours
8 - 12 months	7 - 8	q 8 hours

Content of Infant Formulas

Specific formula	Kcal/oz	Carbohydrate %kcal	Carbohydrate type	Protein g/100 kcal	Protein type	Fat g/100 kcal	Fat Type[1]	Ca:P mg	Na:K:meq 100 kcal	Iron mg[2] in 100 kcal	Use Indication
breast milk	22	38	lactose	1.1	human	3.9	human	43:24	0.8 : 1.1	0.03	normal lactation
cow's milk	19	48	lactose	34	bovine	34	butterfat	high	21:39	0.5	>1y, normal GI
Similac	20	43	lactose	1.5	bovine	3.6	soy coconut	50:38	0.8:1.8	0.3 (1.2)	normal GI tract
Enfamil	20	41	lactose	3.8	bovine	1.5	* + palm	53:36	0.8:1.9	0.3 (1.3)	normal GI tract
Similac PM 60:40	20	41	lactose	1.6	bovine	3.8	soy coconut	38:19	0.7:1.5	0.15	infants requiring low Ca+P levels
Alimentum	20	41	sucrose tapioca	1.9	casein	3.8	MCT, soy safflower	71:51	1.3:2	1.2	food allergy, fat-protein malab.
Neocate	21	47	safflower	2.0	free amino acids	3.2	corn, soy safflower	49:35	0.8:1.6	1.1	severe food allergies
ProSobee	20	40	corn syrup solids	2.0	soy methionin	3.5	soy coconut	63:49	1:2:1	1.3	cow milk allergy, lactose malab., galactosemia
Isomil	20	40	corn syrup sucrose	1.8	soy methionin	3.7	palm, soy coconut	71:51	1.3:1.9	1.2	see Prosobee
Isomil SF	20	40	glucose polymers	1.8	soy methionin	3.6	soy coconut	70:50	1.3:1.8	1.2	see Prosobee
Progestimil	20	41	corn syrup tapioca	1.9	casein amino acid	3.8	corn MCT's	63:42	1.1:1.9	1.3	food allergy, fat-protein malab.
Nutramigen	20	44	corn syrup	1.9	*	3.3	see Isomil	63:42	1.4:1.9	1.3	food allergy
Portagen	20	46	corn syrup sucrose	1.9	sodium caseinate	3.1	corn MCT's	63:47	1.6:2.1	1.3	fat malabsorption

[1]MCT's = medium-chain triglycerides. [2]Iron in parentheses is that in the iron fortified formula for particular brand.

Orthopedics

Differential of Painful Hip (or Limp)

Features	Toxic synovitis	Legg-Calve Perthes	Septic arthritis	Slipped capital femoral epiphysis
Age (yrs)	1½ -12	4-9	< 2, but any age	8-16
Sex (M:F)	3:2	5:1	1:1	2:1
History	prior URI	minimally painful limp	acute fever, ± preceding URI	obesity in 88%
Physical exam	limited hip abduction and rotation	limited hip abduction	hip often held flexed and abducted	Trendelenberg gait, hip externally rotates with flexion
X-rays	enlargement of medial joint space	subchondral lucency in subcortical femoral head	distended joint space, femoral head laterally subluxed	line along superior aspect femoral neck transects <20% epiphysis
Ultrasound	effusion ~90%	no effusion	effusion	no effusion
WBC/ESR	normal	normal	elevated	normal

All 4 disorders above have abnormal bone scans. 20% of children < 5 yo with acute limp have a fracture (typically tibia/fibula if < 2 yo). Other serious disorders to consider: Discitis/osteomyelitis (refusal to walk or slow cautious walk), puncture wound of foot with retained foreign body, neoplasms, and JRA (the knee is often the first joint involved and patients often are 2-3 years old at presentation).

Criteria for Ordering Knee and Ankle Radiographs in the ED

Knee criteria	Ankle Criteria
• Inability to flex 90° or • Inability to bear weight in the emergency department (ED)	• Inability to bear weight immediately after injury or • Inability to take 4 steps in the ED or • Tenderness along the inferior or posterior edge of either malleolus

Presence of any criteria above was 100% sensitive in detecting fractures. However, confidence intervals for sensitivity were 72-100% for knee, & 77-100% for ankle fractures.

Pediatr Emerg Care 1998; 186.   *Arch Pediatr Adoles Med* 1995; 149: 255.

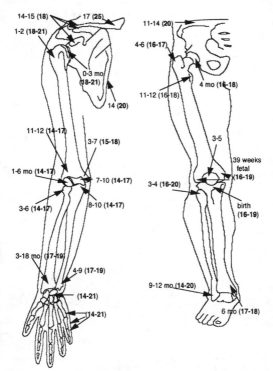

Normal type – Age of onset of secondary ossification centers.
(Bold type in parenthesis) – Age of physeal closure.
All ages are in years unless otherwise specified.

Salter-Harris/Ogden-Harris Physeal Fracture Classification

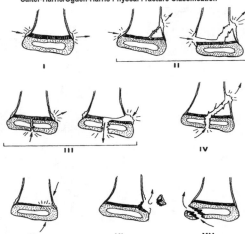

used with permission Strange GR.*Pediatric Emergency Medicine*. A comprehensive study guide. McGraw Hill 1996.

Salter I	Complete separation of the epiphysis and most of physis from metaphysis due to shearing force in infant/neonate. Usually no long term growth problems (except distal/proximal femur, proximal radius, and proximal tibia - can prematurely close with growth arrest)
Salter II	Fracture line extends along physis into metaphysis. Usually > 10 yr. Generally have good prognosis.
Salter III	Fracture line extends physis through epiphysis to articular surface.
Salter IV	Fracture at articular surface crosses epiphysis to metaphysis. Most III and IV injuries will require exact reduction and orthopedic consult.
Salter V	Longitudinal compression of growth plate.
Ogden VI	Peripheral shear to borders of growth plate.
Ogden VII	Intraarticular epiphyseal injury, ligament pulling off distal epiphysis.
Ogden VIII	Fracture through metaphysis with circulation disruption.
Ogden IX	Fracture with loss of periosteum.

Respiratory Disorders

Reference Values (PEFR[1]) for Spirometry

Age	6 years		8 years		10 years		12 years		14 years	
Sex	M[2]	F[3]	M	F	M	F	M	F	M	F
Height (in) 44	99	149	119	168	139	186	159	205	178	224
48	146	179	166	197	186	216	206	235	226	254
52	194	208	214	227	234	246	254	265	274	283
56	241	235	261	256	281	275	301	295	321	314
60	289	268	309	287	329	305	349	324	369	343
64	336	297	356	316	376	335	396	354	416	373
68	384	327	404	346	424	365	444	384	464	403
72	431	357	451	376	471	395	491	414	511	432

[1]PEFR = peak expiratory flow rate. [2]M - male, [3]F – female.

*Ann Rev Resp Dis*1983; 127: 725.

Severity of Asthma Exacerbation (NIH 1997)

Feature	Mild	Moderate	Severe	Pre-Arrest
Breathless	walking	talking	at rest	
Position	can lie down	prefers sitting	sits upright	
Talking	sentences	phrases	words	
Alertness	may be agitated	usually agitated	usually agitated	drowsy/confused
Respiratory rate	Increased	Increased	Rapid	
Acc. muscles	usually not	common	usually	
Wheeze	end expiratory	all expiration	insp.+expiratory	absent wheeze
Pulse	normal	elevated	elevated	bradycardia
Pulsus para.	< 10 mm Hg	10-20 mm Hg	20-40 mm Hg	may be absent
PEFR	> 80%	50-80%	< 50%	
Pao_2 on air	normal	> 60 mm Hg	< 60 mm Hg	
PaCO_2	< 42 mm Hg	< 42 mm Hg	≥ 42 mm Hg	
O_2 sat. room air	> 95%	91-95%	< 91%	

Ann Emerg Med 1998; 31: 579.

Clinical Asthma Score

Feature	0[1]	1	2
po_2 (mm Hg) [1]	70-100 room air	< 70 room air	< 70 on 40% Fio_2
Cyanosis	None	room air	on 40% Fio_2
Inspiratory sounds	Normal	Unequal	Diminished
Accessory muscles	None	Moderate	Maximal
Expiratory wheezing	None	Moderate	Marked
Mental status	Normal	Depressed	Coma

[1]May substitute O_2 saturation of 91% for pO_2 of 70 mm Hg. *Am J Dis Child 1972; 123: 227.*
A total score ≥ 5 = impending respiratory failure, ≥ 7 = existing respiratory failure.

Criteria associated with severe disease and high likelihood of admission to hospital	• Pretreatment PEFR and FEV1 < 25% predicted • Pulsus paradoxicus > 10 mm Hg on presentation • Failure of PEFR to rise > 15% after treatment • Posttreatment PEFR and FEV1 < 60% predicted or PO_2 <60-80, PCO_2 > 40-45, pH <7.35, or SaO_2 <93%

Guidelines for ED Management of Asthma (NIH 1997)

History, examination, O_2 saturation, peak flow (PEFR) or FEV1

FEV1 or PEFR > 50%
- β_2 agonist by MDI or neb. X 3 1st hr
- O_2 to keep sat. ≥ 90 %
- Oral steroids if no immediate response

FEV1 or PEFR < 50%
- High dose β_2 agonist + anticholinergic neb q 20 min or continue X 1 hr
- O_2 to keep sat. ≥ 90 %
- Oral steroids

Impending arrest
- Intubation + ventilate with 100%
- β_2 agonist + anticholinergic neb.
- IV steroids

Repeat exam, PEFR, O_2 saturation as needed

Admit to ICU (see below)

Moderate exacerbation
- PEFR 50-80% of predicted best
- Moderate symptoms
- Inhaled β_2 agonists q 60 minutes
- Oral or increased inhaled steroids
- Treat 1-3 hours, if improvement

Severe exacerbation
- PEFR < 50% of predicted best
- Severe rest symptoms, high risk
- No improvement after initial treatment
- Inhaled β_2 agonists q hr or continuous + inhaled anticholinergics
- O_2 and systemic steroids

Good response
- PEFR ≥ 70%, sustain response 60 minutes
- Normal exam

Incomplete response
- PEFR ≥ 50% , < 70%
- Mild to moderate symptoms

Poor response
- PEFR < 50%
- pCO_2 ≥ 42 mm Hg
- Severe symptoms

OR ↓ (individualize)

Discharge home
- Continue inhaled β_2 agonists + oral steroid
- Patient education regarding medicines, review plan, follow-up

Admit to hospital
- Inhaled β_2 agonist and anticholinergic
- Oral or IV steroid
- O_2 to keep sat. ≥ 90 %
- Follow PEFR,HR,O_2sat

Admit to ICU
- Inhaled β_2 agonist hourly or continuous
- IV steroids
- Oxygen
- Possible intubation

NIH Guidelines for Diagnosis/Management of Asthma *Ann Emerg Med* 1998; 31: 579.

Parenteral Agents for Treating Acute Asthma

Agent	Dose (max dose)	Frequency	Comments
epinephrine 1:1000	0.01 mg/kg SC (0.4ml)	q 20 minutes	nonselective α,β agonist
Sus-Phrine 1:200	0.005 ml/kg SC (0.2ml)	single dose	long acting epinephrine
ketamine	1-2 mg/kg IV	-	primarily if intubated
magnesium sulfate	25 mg/kg IV (2 g)	-	administer over 15 min
methylprednisolone	1-2 mg/kg IV	q 6 hours	-
terbutaline (1mg/ml)	0.01 mg/kg SC	q 20 minutes	more β selective than epi
terbutaline	2 ug/kg IV over 5min, then 4.5 ug/kg/h IV	load over 5 min 4.5 ug/kg/hour	monitor in ICU , reduce dose 50% if theophylline
theophylline	5.6mg/kg + 0.3-1mg/kg/h		Loading + maintenance

Inhaled Asthma Medications

Agent	Dose/Frequency[1]	Comments
albuterol 0.05% (*Ventolin*)	Neb: 0.5-1ml in 2.5 ml NS q30min or continuous, then 2 puffs q 4h (MDI)	β agonist (more selective β_2 than isoetharine, and metaproterenol)
atropine (1mg/ml)	0.1-0.3 ml/kg q30 minX2	more tachycardia than β agonists
beclomethasone (*Vanceril*)	2-4 puffs bid-qid	not approved < 6 yr
cromolyn (*Intal*)	Neb: 20 mg bid or 2 puffs bid-qid (MDI)	maintenance only, $\pm$ not useful acutely
flunisolide(*Aerobid*)	2 puffs bid (MDI)	not approved < 6 yo
ipratropium (*Atrovent*)	Neb: 500 ug q 6-8h 2 puffs tid-qid (MDI)	anticholinergic with longer onset of action than most β agonists
isoetharine 1% (*Bronkosol*)	Neb: 0.25-0.5 ml q 20 min, then q 4-6 h	poor β_2 selectivity
metaproterenol (*Alupent*)	0.25-.5 mg/kg/dose q4-6	less β_2 selective, max dose 15 mg
salmeterol (*Serevent*)	2 puffs bid (MDI)	long acting β agonist, maintenance only, approved > 11 yr

[1]Nebulizer (mixed with 2.5 ml NS) unless otherwise stated, MDI - metered dose inhaler.

Oral Asthma Medications

Agent	Preparation	Dose	Comment
albuterol (*Ventolin*)	2 mg/5ml Tabs: 2,4 mg	0.10-0.15 mg/kg per dose (tid-qid)	β agonist
metaproterenol (*Alupent*)	10 mg/5ml Tabs: 10, 20 mg	2 mg/kg/day (qid)	β agonist
prednisolone-*Prelone* 15/5 *Pediapred* 5/5	15 mg/5ml; 5 mg/5ml Tabs: 5 mg	1-2 mg/kg/day	steroid, if treat 5-7 d no taper needed
prednisone (*LiquidPred*)	5 mg/5ml; Tabs: 1, 2.5, 5, 10, 20, 50	1-2 mg/kg/day	" "
montelukast (*Singulair*) [leukotriene inhibitor]	Tabs: 5, 10 mg	5 mg qhs 6-14 y 10 mg qhs > 14 y	prophylactic, not approved < 6 years

Comparison of Stridorous Upper Airway Diseases in Children

Feature	Croup	Bacterial Tracheitis	Epiglottitis
Age range (years)	0.3-3.0	5-10	2-8
Prodrome	days	hours to days	minutes to hours
Temperature	low grade	often > 101ºF	often > 101ºF
Radiography	steeple sign	exudate in trachea	thumb sign, ratios[1]
Etiology	parainfluenza	staph aureus/strep A	H. influenzae type b
Barky cough	yes	yes	no
Drooling	no	no	yes
Appear toxic	no	yes	yes
Intubation? ICU?	no	yes	yes
Antibiotics	no	yes	yes

[1] 3 calculations are reported as 100% sensitive and specific for epiglottitis: AEW/C3W>.35, EW/C3W>0.50, & EW/EH>0.6: EW=epiglottic width, EH=epiglottic height, C3W=C3 vertebral width, and AEW=aryepiglottic fold width. Ann Emerg Med 1990; 19: 978

Therapy for croup and post-intubation stridor:

- **Humidified** O_2
- **Dexamethasone** 0.6 mg/kg IM or PO, or oral prednisolone
- **Aerosolized racemic epinephrine** (RE) 0.25-0.50 ml of 2.25% solution diluted 1:8 or standard epinephrine 1 ml of 1:1,000 (cheaper + similar side effects). Improved children treated with RE with no worsening in 3h may be discharged.
- **Aerosolized budesonide** – 2 mg (4 ml) via nebulizer
- **Heliox** – when inhaled may be useful at decreasing airway resistance.

Croup Score (add the 5 elements together)[1]

Feature	0	1	2	3
Color	normal	dusky	cyanotic	cyanotic on O_2
Air movement	normal	mild↓	moderate↓	marked↓
Retractions	none	mild	moderate	severe
Mentation	normal	restless	lethargic	obtunded
Stridor	none	mild	moderate	severe/obstructed

Total score	Severity	Treatment
0-4	mild	cool mist, home care
5-6	mild/moderate	cool mist, admit if <6 months or unreliable family
7-8	moderate	racemic epinephrine, consider steroids, admit most
9-14	severe	racemic epinephrine, steroids, ICU admission
15	terminal	racemic epinephrine, steroids, intubation

[1] Any category with score of 3, classify as severe. Taussig: Am J Dis Child 1975; 129: 790.

Pneumonia

- _Chlamydia_ is seen at 3-16 weeks. 1st rhinorrhea, then staccato cough, ↑RR, rales or wheezing. 95% are afebrile + 50% have concurrent/prior conjunctivitis.
- _Pneumococcus and H flu_ are typically associated with abrupt onset of high fever and dyspnea, and may be preceded by a viral URI.
- _Mycoplasma_ presents with low-grade fever, malaise, headache, and nonproductive cough lasting weeks. It is responsible for 9-21% of school-aged pneumonia, may occur in epidemics, and has little seasonal variation.
- _Tuberculosis_ typically presents with subacute cough, night sweats, ↓ weight.
- _Bordatella pertussis_ mimics chlamydial pneumonitis, but has a paroxysmal, inspiratory 'whoop' (may be absent in those < 6 months). Prolonged coughing attacks may lead to cyanosis, emesis, and anoxia.

Age	Etiology
newborn	Causes include Group B streptococcus, E coli, Listeria, and herpes virus
1-4 months	*Febrile*: pneumococcus, H flu (rare). *Afebrile*: chlamydia, ureaplasma, mycoplasma, pneumocystis, and cytomegalovirus
5 months - 5 years	Viruses (especially RSV) are most common, followed by pneumococcus, Mycoplasma. H flu is now rare. Ratio of viral to bacterial etiology is 5:2.
> 5 years	Mycoplasma followed by pneumococcus

High Yield Indications for Chest Radiography	<ul><li>Tachypnea (the single best predictor of pneumonia)</li><li>Rales (1/3 will have infiltrate), ↓breath sounds</li><li>Stridor, grunting, flaring, retractions, or cyanosis</li><li>Absence of above and presence of wheezing, prolonged expiration or rhonchi with cough have low yield</li></ul>

Emerg Med Reports 1995; 16: 183.

Predictive Value of Respiratory rate In Pneumonia	Age	Respiratory rate[1]	Sensitivity	NPV[2]
	0-5 months	≥ 59	83%	99%
	6-11 months	≥ 52	67%	98%
	1-2 years	≥ 42	71%	96%

[1]Breaths/min. [2]NPV – negative predictive value = probability of normal CXR if below rate.
Arch Pediatr Adolesc Med 1995; 149: 283.

Indications for Hospital Admission

• Age < 2-3 months	• Toxic appearance
• Lobar infiltrate and < 12 months	• Immunocompromised
• Multilobar, effusion, pneumatocoele	• Unresponsive to oral medications
• Respiratory distress or hypoxia	• Unable to keep down liquids or meds

Antibiotic therapy for pneumonia is detailed on page 61.

Reye's Syndrome

Overview: 70% with Reye's syndrome have had recent URI (e.g., influenza A or B), 15-30% recent varicella, and 2-15% recent diarrhea. Most cases occur during peak influenza period of January to March. 0.05% patients with influenza B + 0.003% with influenza A develop Reye's. Reye's is associated with isopropyl alcohol, lead, methyl bromide, insecticides, insect repellent, aflatoxin, phenothiazines, and aspirin use. Patients develop inflammation and edema of the liver and brain.

Clinical Features
• Vomiting 1 week after prodromal illness
• Headache, lethargy, seizures (30%)
• Absent meningeal signs
• Younger children (less vomiting, less prodrome)
• Hepatomegaly (within 24-48 hours of diagnosis)

Clinical Stage	Signs and Symptoms
0	alert, vomiting, liver dysfunction
I	lethargic, vomiting, liver dysfunction
II	delirious, combative
III	obtunded, decorticate, reactive pupils, possible seizures
IV	obtunded, decerebrate, unreactive pupils
V	flaccid, areflexic, apneic, liver function often normalized

Labs in Reye's Syndrome	Treatment of Reye's Syndrome

• ↑ AST/ALT (≥ 2X normal) – most sensitive screening test
• ↑ ammonia (≥ 1.5 normal) – rises early and normalizes quickly
• → bilirubin (< 3 mg/dl)
• ↓ glucose (70-80% of infants)
• ↓pCO_2, ↓CO_2
• ↑creatinine and↑BUN in 30-40%
• ↑amylase (pancreatitis in 9%)
	• D_{10}.9NS keep glucose150-200 mg/dl
	• Keep fluids at 2/3 maintenance rate
	• If ≥ Stage II consider:
	  - intubation, elevate head of bed
	   (all III, and II if ammonia > 300)
	  - deep sedation
	  - cerebral pressure monitoring
	  - mannitol 0.5-1 g/kg IV q 6 h
	  - lactulose 0.3g/kg PO/NG q 6 h

Prognosis: Risk of progression from stage I to coma is high with elevated transaminases, PT (>3 seconds above normal), or ammonia (>100 µg/dl). Poor prognosis at stage II-IV level is indicated by age < 1 year, ammonia 6 X normal, CK 10 X normal, rapid progression, or seizures in stage III. Most recover without sequelae. 10% develop chronic neurologic problems (e.g., seizure disorder, encephalopathy).

Surgical Abdominal Disorders

Most Common Etiologies of Abdominal Pain in Children Presenting to a Pediatric ED *Pediatr Emerg Care 1992;8:126*	Nonspecific pain	36%	Pharyngitis	6%
	Gastroenteritis	16%	Viral illness	3%
	Appendicitis	8%	Pneumonia	2%
	Constipation	7%	Otitis Media	2%
	Urinary infection	6%	Other disease	14%

High Yield Criteria for Ordering Plain Xrays in Children	The presence any criteria is 93-100% sensitive in detecting plain Xrays that are diagnostic or suggestive of major surgical disease. If no criteria are present, plain films have < 1% probability of revealing a surgical disorder. Plain films are normal in 50% and misleading in 2% with surgical disease.
• prior abdominal surgery, • peritoneal signs, • foreign body ingestion, • abdominal distention, or • abnormal bowel sounds	

Ann Emerg Med 1992; 21:1423.

Radiologic Studies in Surgical Abdominal Disorders

Disorder	Radiologic adjunct	Key features
Appendicitis	Ultrasound	Multiple pediatric studies with sensitivity of 85-90%. Less accurate if perforated/gangrenous
	Computerized tomography	No pediatric studies, 5 adult studies with 90-100% sensitivity in uncomplicated appendicitis
Hirschprung's	Barium enema	Shows normal rectum, dilated proximal colon
Intussus-ception	Ultrasound	98% sensitive in limited studies
	Barium or air contrast enema	Air contrast enema is standard for diagnosis with 60-90% successful reduction rate
Meckel's	Technetium scan	95% sensitive (esp. if given with cimetidine) False negatives occur if little gastric mucosa
Malrotation	Ultrasonography	May show bowel wall edema, intraluminal fluid
	UGI series	Shows obstruction at 3rd portion duodenum
Pyloric stenosis	Ultrasound	89-95% sensitive
	UGI series	95% sensitive, risks aspiration, delays surgery

Pediatr Emerg Med Reports 1997; 2: 111.

Appendicitis

Risk of Appendicitis MANTRELS scoring system[1]		

Item	Score
Migration of pain to RLQ	1
Anorexia or acetone in urine	1
Nausea with vomiting	1
Tenderness in right low quadrant	2
Rebound tenderness	1
Elevated temperature > 100.4 F	1
Leukocytosis; WBC > 10,500	2
Shift of WBC's; >75% neutrophils	1

Total	Action
≥ 7	Candidates for surgery
4-6	Serial exams or further testing (CT or US)
< 4	Extremely low probability of appendicitis

[1] This score is <u>unreliable</u> in younger children and infants.   *Resident Staff Phys 1995; 11-18.*

Annular pancreas is associated with malrotation and Downs syndrome. Bilious vomiting is the hallmark, as the obstruction is distal to the Ampulla of Vater.

Gastric volvulus A torsion ≤ 180 degrees produces a partial obstruction with or without vomiting which may not lead to vascular compromise. Torsion > 180 degrees causes Borchardt's triad: (1) retching, (2) acute epigastric pain, (3) distention with inability to pass a NG. Respiratory distress or GI bleeding occur.

Hirschsprung's Disease (congenital megacolon): Congenital absence of parasympathetic ganglion cells in Auerbach's plexus (myenteric) and Meissner's (submucosal) plexus in the intestine, causing un-coordinated intestinal motility. In 80-90%, involvement is limited to rectum and rectosigmoid colon including the internal anal sphincter. Hirschsprung's is noted in 1/5,000 births and is more common in males and Down's syndrome. In newborns, it may present as complete obstruction or delayed passage of meconium with mild constipation. Most affected infants are full term. If left untreated, failure to thrive will be noted, with ill appearance, malnourishment, or chronic constipation. The most serious complication is the development of ulcerative enterocolitis, which may be lethal. In this complication, elevated luminal pressures in the proximal normal colon inhibit total colonic blood flow and shunt blood away from the mucosa. Bowel wall edema, mucosal necrosis and sepsis occur. Diagnosis is made by barium enema (BE). If BE is nondiagnostic, consider rectal biopsy with acetylcholinesterase histochemistry on mucosa and submucosal biopsy specimens. Children with functional constipation are generally healthy appearing with bowel troubles beginning around age 2 years or the time of toilet training, have stool in rectal vault, & fecal soiling. Hirschsprung's patients are generally younger, have empty rectal vault, and no fecal soiling.

Incarcerated hernias Manual reduction may be useful regardless of time and may still work if obstruction is present. Avoid manual reduction if peritonitis, unstable vitals, significant erythema or other sign of strangulation. Bimanual abdominal/rectal exam may identify mass between fingers, a finding absent in spermatic cord hydrocele. Palpation of the inguinal region may reveal a dilated external ring or a silk glove sign (smoothness felt as if 2 pieces of silk are being rubbed together when rolling the spermatic cord in a direction perpendicular to the inguinal canal).

Intussusception A telescoping of 1 intestinal segment into adjacent segment. It is the leading cause of intestinal obstruction between 3 months and 6 years. Average age is 7-8 months, with 80% < 2 years old. Origin is unknown in 90-95% unless < 1 month or > 3 years where a lead point (e.g., tumor) may be found.

Predisposing Conditions

- Henoch Schonlein Purpura (HSP) is noted in 3% of cases. None are reducible.
- Cystic fibrosis - Barium enema reduction is unlikely in Cystic fibrosis.
- Peutz Jehger syndrome is a rare cause of intussusception in older children.
- Intestinal lymphosarcoma can cause a chronic non-strangulating intussusception and should be suspected in all cases of intussusception older than 6 years.
- Post-operative - after retroperitoneal dissection (e.g., Wilm's tumor).

Clinical features: A previously well infant who cries out in paroxysms of pain, draws up both legs and vomits. Passage of a formed or liquid stool provides relief with recurrence of symptoms in 20-60 minutes. Within hours, child may become lethargic with passage of blood per rectum. Exam may reveal abdominal distention and/or a sausage shaped abdominal mass, often in RUQ.

Diagnosis/Treatment: X-ray may show the head of the intussusception projecting into the air filled colon in up to 60%. US may be diagnostic with classic "bulls eye" appearance in > 95%. BE or air-contrast enema reduces intussusception in 60-90%. An enema is often therapeutic but should be avoided if shock, peritoneal signs, perforation, or high grade obstruction.

Protocol for Contrast Reduction of Intussusception

1. Consult surgeon and prepare operating room.
2. Place nasogastric tube, and restore fluid status to normal via IV route.
3. Insert non-lubricated 20-24F Foley into rectum, inflate balloon 5-10 ml and pull down against levators. Compress buttocks and tape together, wrap legs.
4. Allow contrast agent to flow by gravity into colon from height of <1 meter.
5. DO NOT palpate abdomen during procedure and use fluoroscope intermittently.
6. Stop attempt if contrast column is stationary and outline unchanged for 10 min.
7. Reduction is complete when there is (1) free flow of barium or air into small bowel, (2) expulsion of feces and flatus with contrast, (3) disappearance of mass, or (4) improvement in the child's condition.

Malrotation and midgut volvulus are characterized by sudden vomiting which may be bilious (malrotation until proven otherwise), bloody or coffee ground appearance. Stool usually contains blood. An upper GI series can be diagnostic, but immediate surgery should be considered instead if there is evidence of complete obstruction.

Meckel's diverticulum arises from failure of omphalomesenteric duct to close. It is found in 2% of the population within 2 feet (100 cm) of the ileocecal valve. Most individuals remain asymptomatic, with complications developing at some point in 23-40%. Complications usually occur prior to 10-30 years of age. Obstruction is most common presentation if intussusception is also present. Bleeding can be the major manifestation, especially in children < 2 years old. Meckel's account for 50% of lower GI bleeding in this age range. Bleeding is usually painless and sudden. Inflammation (e.g., diverticulitis) may present like appendicitis in 20%, and is most common around age 8 years. Up to 50% perforate before surgery. Diagnosis of Meckel's is made with a Technetium (Tc99 or "Meckel's") scan, which has a sensitivity of 75-100% and a specificity of 80%. A higher incidence of true positives occur if cimetidine is given 24h prior to the scan, if the clinical condition permits this delay. By blocking histamine, cimetidine prevents secretion and increases concentration of Tc from gastric mucosa. BE is only diagnostic in 4-20% of cases.

Necrotizing enterocolitis (NEC) occurs in premature infants in NICU's. Strictures develop within 6 months of birth in 11-36% of NEC cases, and may result in abdominal pain or bowel obstruction.

Post-operative adhesive small bowel obstruction causes 7% of intestinal obstructions in children. 2% of laparotomy patients will develop this complication.

Pyloric Stenosis (PS) occurs in 1/3,000 infants with males affected more than females. PS is rare in premature infants and more common in 1st born males, advanced maternal primagravida age, and use of bendectin. 21% have anomalies of the upper urinary tract. Symptoms classically begin at 2-3 weeks, although PS can be seen up to 5 months. *Clinical features*: Mild non-bilious vomiting during or after feeding, with development of projectile vomiting ~ 1 week later. Patients are hungry and may exhibit poor weight gain. *Physical Examination*: Dehydration is typical. Abdominal examination may reveal peristaltic waves or a palpable "olive" in 70-95%. If evacuation of the stomach with a #10-12F NG tube reveals ≥ 90-150 ml of fluid, then a gastric outlet obstruction is likely. Hypochloremic metabolic alkalosis may be noted. *Diagnosis*: Ultrasonography or an UGI series are > 95% sensitive.

Toxins that Affect Vitals Signs and Physical Examination

Hypotension			Hypertension
ACE inhibitors	Antidepressants	Nitroprusside	Amphetamines
α & β antagonists	Disulfuram	Opioids	Anticholinergics
Anticholinergics	Ethanol, methanol	Organophosphates	Cocaine, Lead
Arsenic (acutely)	Iron, Isopropanol	Phenothiazines	MAO inhibitors
Ca^{+2} channel block	Mercury	Sedatives	Phencyclidine
Clonidine, cyanide	Nitrates	Theophylline	Sympathomemetics

Tachycardia		Bradycardia	
Amphetamines	Ethylene glycol, iron	Antidysrhythmics	
Anticholinergics	Organophosphates	α agonists, β antagonists	
Arsenic (acutely)	Phencyclidine	Ca^{+2} channel blockers	
Antidepressants	Phenothiazines	Digitalis, opioids	
Digitalis, disulfuram	Theophylline	Organophosphates	

Tachypnea		Bradypnea	
Ethylene glycol	Salicylates	Barbiturates	Isopropanol
Methanol	Sympathomimetics	Botulism	Opioids
Nicotine	Theophylline	Clonidine	Organophosphates
Organophosphates		Ethanol	Sedatives

Hyperthermia		Hypothermia
Amphetamines	Phencyclidine	Carbon monoxide
Anticholinergics	Phenothiazines	Ethanol
Arsenic (acute)	Salicylates	Hypoglycemic agents
Cocaine	Sedative-hypnotics	Opioids
Antidepressants	Theophylline	Phenothiazines
LSD	Thyroxine	Sedative-hypnotics

Mydriasis (pupillodilation)		Miosis (pupilloconstriction)	
Anticholinergics	Amphetamines	Anticholinesterase	Clonidine
Antihistamines	Cocaine	Opioids	Coma from barbit-
Antidepressants	Sympathomimetics	Nicotine	urates, benzodi-
Anoxia (any cause)	Drug withdrawal	Pilocarpine	azepines, ethanol

Toxins that Cause Seizures

Antidepressants	Cocaine, camphor	INH, Lead, Lithium	Organophosphates
β blockers	Ethanol withdrawal	PCP, theophylline	Sympathomimetics

[1] All agents causing ↓BP, fever, hypoglycemia and CNS bleeding can cause seizures.

Poisoning (Toxidromes)

Syndrome	Toxin	Manifestations
anticho-linergic	*Natural*: belladonna alkaloids, atropine, homatropine, amanita muscurina. *Synthetics*: cyclopentolate, dicyclomine, tropicanimide, antihistamines, tricyclics, phenothiazines	*Peripheral antimuscarinic*: dry skin, thirst, blurred vision, mydriasis, ↑ pulse, ↑BP, red rash, ↑temperature, abdominal distention, urine retention. *Central symptoms*: delirium, ataxia, cardiovascular collapse, seizures
acetyl-cholines-terase inhibition	insecticides (organophosphates, carbamates)	*Muscarinic effects* (SLUDGE): salivation, lacrimation, urination, defecation, GI upset, emesis. Also ↓or↑ pulse and BP, miosis. *Nicotinic effects*: ↑pulse, muscle fasciculations, weakness, paralysis, ↓respirations, sympathetic stimulation. *Central effects*: anxiety, ataxia, seizure, coma, ↓respirations, cardiovascular collapse
choli-nergic	acetylcholine, betelnut, bethanechol, clitocybe, methacholine, pilocarpine	see *muscarinic* and *nicotinic* effects above
extra-pyramidal	haloperidol, phenothiazines	*Parkinsonism*: dysphonia, rigidity, tremor, torticollis, opisthotonis
hemoglo-binopathy	carbon monoxide, methemoglobin	headache, nausea, vomiting, dizziness, coma, seizures, cyanosis, cutaneous bullae, "chocolate" blood with methemoglobinemia
metal fume fever	iron, magnesium, mercury, nickel, zinc, cadmium, copper	chills, fever, muscle pain, headache, fatigue, weakness
narcotic	morphine, dextromethorphan, heroin, fentanyl, meperidine, propoxyphene, codeine, diphenoxylate	CNS depression, miosis (except meperidine), ↓respirations, ↓BP, seizures (with propoxyphene)
sympatho-mimetic	aminophylline, amphetamines, cocaine, ephedrine, caffeine, methylphenidate	CNS excitation, seizures, ↑pulse, ↑BP (↓BP with caffeine)
with-drawal syndrome	alcohol, barbiturates, benzodiazepines, cocaine, narcotics, opioids	diarrhea, mydriasis, piloerection, ↑BP, ↑pulse, insomnia, lacrimation, cramps, yawning, hallucinations

Poisoning Antidotes and Treatments

Toxin	Antidote	Other considerations
acetamino-phen	n-acetylcysteine see page 95 for dose	very effective if used within 8h, may be helpful up to 72h
β-blockers	glucagon 50-150 µg/kg IV, SC, or IM	glucagon may help reverse ↓pulse and ↓BP
Ca^{+2}channel blockers	CaCl$_2$ (10%) 0.3 ml/kg IV, glucagon-see β blocker dose	glucagon may help reverse ↓pulse and ↓BP
cyanide	*Lilly Cyanide Kit* (amyl nitrate, sodium nitrite, and sodium thiosulfate)	Treatment induces methemo-globinemia and ↓BP. Sodium thiocyanate is excreted in urine.
digoxin	digoxin Fab fragments	see page 100 for dose
ethylene glycol	ethanol 1 ml/kg of 100% ethanol IV in glucose solution dialysis, fomepizole (*Antizol*)	ethanol competes for alcohol dehydrogenase, goal is an ethanol level of 0.1 g/dl 15 mg/kg X 1, 10 mg/kg q 12 X 4
isoniazid	pyridoxine up to 25 mg/kg IV	reverses seizures
methanol	ethanol, dialysis (± *Antizol*)	also thiamine and folate
nitrites	methylene blue (0.2 ml/kg of 1% solution IV over 5 min)	consider exchange transfusion if severe methemoglobinemia
opiates	naloxone 0.4-2.0 mg IV	diphenoxylate and propoxyphene may require higher doses
organo-phosphates, carbamates	atropine 0.05 mg/kg IV pralidoxime (PAM)	exceptionally high atropine doses may be necessary; PAM doesn't work for carbamate toxicity
salicylates	dialysis, or sodium bicarbonate 1 mEq/kg IV	goal of alkaline diuresis is urine pH of 7.50-7.55
tricyclic anti-depressants	sodium bicarbonate 1 mEq/kg IV	goal is serum pH of 7.50-7.55 to alter protein binding

Radio-opaque ingestions (CHIPES)	Drugs Cleared by Hemodialysis[1]	
• **C**hloral hydrate and Chlorinated hydrocarbons	• Salicylates	• Isopropyl alcohol
• **H**eavy metals (arsenic, Pb, mercury) health food (bone meal, vitamins)	• Ethylene glycol	• Chloral hydrate
	• Methanol	• Lithium
• **I**odides, iron	• Bromide	
• **P**otassium, psychotropics (e.g. phenothiazines, antidepressants)	**Drugs cleared by Hemoperfusion[1]**	
	• Barbiturates (e.g. phenobarbital)	
• **E**nteric coated tabs (KCl, salicylates)	• Theophylline	
• **S**olvents (chloroform, CCl$_4$)	• Phenytoin	
	• Possibly digoxin	

[1] Consult local poison center for more detail concerning latest recommendations

General Approach to the Poisoned Child

• Treat airway, breathing and BP	• Administer dextrose 2-4 ml/kg of D_{25}
• Insert IV and apply cardiac monitor	if ≤ 2, 50 ml of D_{50}, > 2 years.
• Apply pulse oximeter, administer O_2	• Administer naloxone 2 mg IV

Charcoal

Initial dose is 1 g/kg PO or per NG mixed with cathartic such as sorbitol

Contraindications	Drugs Cleared by Multi-dose Charcoal[1]
• Caustics (acids, alkalis)	theophylline, phenobarbital, digoxin,
• Ileus, bowel obstruction	dextropropoxyphene, nadolol, phenytoin,
• Drugs bound poorly by charcoal (arsenic, bromide, K^+, toxic alcohols, heavy metals [iron, iodide, lithium])	diazepam, tricyclic antidepressants, chlorpropamide, nonsteroidals, and salicylates

[1] Administer repeat charcoal doses q 3-4 hours (use cathartic only for 1st dose).

Cathartics

Cathartics theoretically help by ↑ fecal elimination of charcoal-bound toxins, and preventing concretions. Monitor electrolytes closely with their use.	Cathartic choices
	• Sorbitol (35%) – 1 g/kg PO or NG
	• Magnesium citrate 4 ml/kg PO or NG
	• Na^+ or $MgSO_4$ – 250 mg/kg PO or NG

Ipecac

There are no absolute indications for use and some experts recommend never using in the ED. Ipecac delays charcoal administration, & has many adverse effects.

Age	1st dose	Repeat	Absolute contraindications to ipecac
<6 mo	do not use	do not use	• Pure caustics or hydrocarbons
6-12 mo	5-10 ml	in 30 min	• Drugs that cause seizures, ↓mental status, ↓HR, or ↓respirations
1-12 yrs	15-30 ml	in 30 min	
>12 yrs	30 ml	in 30 min	• Nontoxic ingestions

Gastric lavage

Directions for Lavage in Overdose	Indications
• Use 16-28 French *Ewald* tube	• Dangerous ingestion < 1 hour old
• Lavage stomach with 15 ml/kg NS aliquots until return is clear	• Toxins that slow GI transit
	• Toxins with possible rapid onset seizure, or ↓mental status
• Protect the airway with endotracheal intubation if there is an absent gag reflex, or altered mental status	• Toxins poorly bound by charcoal
	Contraindications
• Monitor total input and output from the *Ewald* tube	• Caustics (acids, alkalis), solvents (hydrocarbons), nontoxic ingestions

Whole bowel irrigation

Administration	Indications
• Place NG tube	• Iron, zinc, sustained release meds
• Administer polyethylene glycol (*Go-Litely*) at 25-40 ml/kg/h[1]	• Ingested crack vials or drug packets
	Contraindications
• Stop when objects recovered or	• CNS or respiratory depression
• Stop when effluent clear	• Ileus, bowel obstruction, perforation

[1] until rectal effluent clear

Acetaminophen

Phase	Time after ingestion	Signs and Symptoms
1	30 min to 24 hours	Asymptomatic, or minor GI irritant effects
2	24-72 hours	Relatively asymptomatic, GI symptoms resolve, possible mild elevation of LFT's or renal failure
3	72-96 hours	Hepatic necrosis with potential jaundice, hepatic encephalopathy, coagulopathy, and renal failure
4	4 days - 2 weeks	Resolution of symptoms or death

Clinical Features-Toxicity Assessment

Ingestion of ≥ 140 mg/kg is potentially toxic. Obtain acetaminophen level ≥ 4h after acute ingestion and plot on the Rumack-Matthews nomogram. A 4h level ≥ 140 µg/ml indicates the need for n-acetylcysteine. On nomogram (page 96), levels above dotted line (--------) indicate probable risk, while levels above bottom solid line (____) indicate possible risk of toxicity. If time from ingestion unknown, obtain level at time 0 and 4 h later to calculate half-life. If half-life is > 4 h, administer antidote.

Treatment

Decontamination	• Charcoal if toxic co-ingestant or waiting for tylenol level.
	• Increase *Mucomyst* dose by 20% if charcoal administered.
N-acetylcysteine *Mucomyst*	• Assess toxicity based on nomogram.
	• If drug level will return in < 8 hours, treatment can be delayed until level known. *Mucomyst* prevents 100% of toxicity if administered < 8 hours from ingestion. If level will return > 8 hours and ≥140 mg/kg ingested, administer 1st dose of *Mucomyst*. *Mucomyst* is definitely useful up to 24 hours after ingestion, with possible utility up to 72 hours.
	• Dose: 140 mg/kg PO, then 70 mg/kg PO q4h X 17 doses.
	• IV *Mucomyst* is used in Europe and not yet FDA approved.

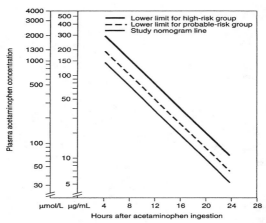

Copyright 1981 American Medical Association. Rumack BH. *Arch Intern Med* 1981; 5: 871.

βeta-Blockers

<u>β1 stimulation</u> - ↑ contraction force + rate, AV node conduction, & renin secretion.
<u>β2 stimulation</u> - blood vessel, bronchi, GI, & GU smooth muscle relaxation.
Propanolol is nonselective, blocking β1 and β2 receptors. Other nonselective β-blockers: nadolol, timolol, pindolol. Selective β1 blockers: metoprolol, atenolol, esmolol, + acebutolol. Pindolol + acebutolol have some β agonist properties.

Clinical Features of β blocker overdose

CNS	• Coma and seizures (esp. with lipid soluble agents – propanolol)
Cardiac	• ↓HR, AV block (1st, 2nd or 3rd), ↑QRS width, ↑T waves, and ST changes
	• ↑HR with pindolol, practolol, and sotalol. ↓BP is common.
	• Congestive heart failure can occur.
Pulmonary	• Bronchospasm and respiratory arrest can occur.
Metabolic	• Hypoglycemia is more common in children compared to adults.

Treatment of β-blocker Toxicity

Option	Recommendations
Gastrointestinal decontamination	• Avoid ipecac. Aspiration & asystole are reported. • Charcoal - repeated doses, ± preceded by gastric lavage
Glucagon	• <u>Indications</u>: ↓HR or BP. • <u>Dose</u>: 50-150 μg/kg + 0.07 mg/kg/h IV
Atropine	• No HR response is suggestive of β-blocker toxicity. Administer 0.02 mg/kg IV prn (maximum of 0.5-1 mg).
Fluid/pressors	• If ↓BP does not respond to NS, administer α + β agonists (epinephrine/norepinephrine) or pure β agonists (dobutamine)
Other options	• Use pacemaker if no response to above. Consider dialysis if atenolol, nadolol, or acebutolol overdose. • Amrinone – 0.75 mg/kg, + 5μg/kg/min IV has +inotropic effect

Calcium Channel Blockers

System	Clinical Features
CNS	• Lethargy, slurred speech, confusion, coma, seizures, ↓respirations
Cardiac	• ↓HR, ↓BP, AV block (1st, 2nd or 3rd), sinus arrest, asystole
GI	• Nausea, vomiting, ileus, obstruction, bowel ischemia/infarction
Metabolic	• Hyperglycemia (esp. verapamil), lactic acidosis

Treatment of Calcium Channel Blocker Toxicity

Option	Recommendations
Gastrointestinal decontamination	• Charcoal ± preceded by gastric lavage. Avoid ipecac. • Whole bowel irrigation if sustained release preparation
Calcium	• Usually ineffective at improving cardiac conduction defects • Primary indication is to reverse hypotension • Administer Ca^{+2} gluconate 0.5-1 ml/kg of 10% solution (max 5 ml) IV over 5 minutes, repeat prn. Alternatively, administer 0.2-0.3 ml/kg of CaCl (10% solution) IV over 5 min.
Glucagon	• Indications: ↓HR or BP. • Dose: 50-150μg/kg + 0.07 mg/kg/h IV
Atropine	• Administer 0.02 mg/kg IV prn symptomatic ↓HR (repeat X 3).
Fluids/pressors	• ↓BP occurs from peripheral vasodilation. Administer NS, then vasoconstrictors (e.g. norepinephrine, neosynephrine or ↑ dose dopamine).
Other options	• Use pacemaker if no response to calcium, glucagon, atropine.

Carbon Monoxide

Carbon monoxide (CO) exposure can occur from fire, catabolism of heme compounds, cigarettes, pollution, ice-surfacing machines, & methylene chloride (dermally absorbed

FIO_2	CO half-life
room air	320 min
100% rebreather	80 min
3 ATM hyperbaric O_2	23 min

paint remover) degradation. CO displaces O_2 off Hb shifting O_2-Hb dissociation curve to left.   CO also binds cytochrome-A, cardiac and skeletal muscle myoglobin.

Clinical Features

CO-Hb level	Typical symptoms at given level of CO toxicity
0-10%	Usually none, $\pm\downarrow$exercise tolerance, $\uparrow$angina, and $\uparrow$claudication
10-20%	Frontal headache, dyspnea with exertion
20-30%	Throbbing headache, dyspnea with exertion, $\downarrow$concentration
30-40%	Severe headache, vomiting, visual changes
40-50%	Confusion, syncope on exertion, myocardial ischemia
50-60%	Collapse, seizures
> 60-70%	Coma and death
Variable	Cherry red skin, visual field defect, homonymous hemianopsia, papilledema, retinal bleed, hearing changes, pulmonary edema. GI upset with vomiting (esp. common < 8 years old)

Assessment of CO Intoxication

CO-Hb levels	Levels are unreliable & may be low in significant intoxication.
Anion gap	Cyanide and lactic acidosis may contribute to anion gap
Saturation gap	Calculated – directly measured arterial O2 saturation. This gap also occurs with cyanide, methemoglobin, & sulfhemoglobin.
EKG	May show changes consistent with myocardial ischemia.
Cardiac enzymes	May be elevated from direct myocardial damage.

Treatment of CO toxicity

Criteria for Admission	Criteria for hyperbaric oxygen
• All with CO-Hb > 15-20% • Pregnancy and CO-Hb > 10% • Acidosis, EKG changes, myocardial ischemia, abnormal neurologic exam or history of unconsciousness • Symptoms persist after 100% O_2 X 3h	• *Absolute*: cyanide toxic, coma, un-concious > 20 min, abnormal neurological examination, abnormal EKG, arrhythmias, or neurologic symptoms after 100% O_2 X 3 h • *Relative*: pregnancy, CO-Hb > 20%.

Clonidine

Clonidine is an α-adrenergic agonist with BP lowering properties, and ability to ameliorate opiate withdrawal symptoms. Tablets of clonidine (*Catapres*), in combination with chlorthalidone (*Combipres*), and transdermal patches (*Catapres-TTS*) are available. Used patches may contain up to 2 mg of active drug. Clonidine is rapidly absorbed from GI tract lowering BP within 30-60 min peaking at 2-4 h. Serum half-life is 12 h (6-24 h). Clonidine lowers BP at the presynaptic α_2-agonist receptors resulting in $\downarrow$ sympathetic outflow. At high doses, it is a peripheral α-agonist and causes $\uparrow$ BP. It is also a CNS depressant.

Clinical Features

General	• Up to 76% of children manifest symptoms by 1 h and 100% by 4h (unless sustained release pill). Symptoms usually last < 24h.
CNS	• Lethargy, coma, recurrent apnea, miosis, hypotonia
Cardiac	• Sinus bradycardia, hypertension (transient), later hypotension
Other	• Hypothermia and pallor

Treatment

Monitor	• Cardiac monitor and pulse oximeter and observe closely for apnea. Apnea often responds to tactile stimulation.
Decontamination	• Charcoal ± gastric lavage. Avoid ipecac.
Atropine	• Indication: bradycardia. Dose: 0.02 mg/kg IV.
Antihypertensives	• Hypertension is usually transient. If needed, use short acting titratable agent (e.g. *Nipride*)
Fluids/pressors	• Treat hypotension with fluids and dopamine prn.
Naloxone	• 0.02 mg/kg IV may reverse CNS but not cardiac/BP effects.

Digoxin

Natural sources: foxglove, oleander, lily of the valley, and the "skin of toads". Therapeutic range - 0.5-2.0 ng/ml. Severe poisoning may not demonstrate $\uparrow$ levels.

Clinical Features – Acute Toxicity	
Digoxin level	Usually markedly elevated (obtain > 6 hours after ingestion)
GI and CNS	Nausea, vomiting, diarrhea, headache, confusion, coma
Cardiac	Supraventricular tachycardia, AV blocks, bradyarrhythmias
Metabolic	Hyperkalemia from inhibition of the Na^+/K^+ ATP pump

Clinical Features – Chronic Toxicity	
Digoxin level	May be normal
History	URI symptoms, on diuretics, renal insufficiency, yellow-green halos
Cardiac	Ventricular arrhythmias are more common than with acute toxicity
Metabolic	Potassium low or normal, magnesium is often low

Treatment of Digoxin Toxicity

• Multi-dose charcoal ± lavage.	• ↑K+: (page 35). Do not use calcium.
• Atropine 0.02 mg/kg for ↓HR	• Avoid cardioversion if possible (pre-
• Ventricular arrhythmia: lidocaine 1	disposes to ventricular fibrillation)
mg/kg IV ± MgSO4 20 mg/kg IV	• Digoxin Fab fragments (*Digibind*)

Indications for Digibind	Total body load digoxin - TBLD estimates
• Ventricular arrhythmias	TBLD (total body load of digoxin) in milligrams =
• Bradyarrhythmias	• [digoxin level[1] (ng/ml) x 5.6 x weight (kg)]÷1000
unresponsive to therapy	• or the total mg ingested if digoxin capsules or
• Ingestion of > 0.1 mg/kg	elixir is ingested
• Digoxin level > 5 ng/ml	• or the total mg ingested X 0.8 if another form of
• Consider if K+ > 5.5 mEq/l	digoxin is ingested

[1] *Chronic ingestions* may have normal to mildly elevated digoxin levels.

Dosing Digibind

- Number of vials to administer = TBLD in mg divided by 0.6
- If ingested quantity unknown consider empiric administration of 2-10 vials
- One 40 mg *Digibind* vial can bind 0.6 mg of digoxin if amount ingested known
- Dilute *Digibind* to 10 mg/ml & administer IV over 20 min. Serum digoxin levels are useless after *Digibind*, as lab assay measures bound + unbound digoxin. These misleading levels may be exceptionally high, as *Digibind* draws digoxin back into the serum. Once bound, digoxin-Fab complex is renally excreted.

Iron Poisoning

Iron Formulations	Elemental Iron	Mechanisms of Iron Toxicity
ferrous gluconate	12%	• Direct GI mucosal damage with hemorrhagic gastritis, bleeding
ferrous sulfate or ferroglycine	20%	• Hepatic necrosis
ferrous fumarate	33%	• Mitochondrial damage
ferrous phosphate	37%	• Venodilation and hypotension
ferrous or ferric pyrophosphate	12%	• 3rd spacing of fluids
ferrocholinate	12%	• Thrombin inhibition- coagulopathy

Clinical Features – Staging of Iron Poisoning

Stage	Time post-ingestion	Findings
I	1-6 hours	Local toxicity: GI bleeding, perforation, diarrhea, and shock due to direct corrosion and vasodilation
II	2-24 hours	Relative stability and resolution: Stage I symptoms resolve
III	4-36 hours	Metabolic disruption: Metabolic acidosis, circulatory collapse, neurologic deterioration, hepatic failure, renal failure, coagulation defects, and third spacing of fluids
IV	2-4 days	Liver failure: Hepatic necrosis
V	2-6 weeks	Late sequelae: GI tract scarring

Clinical Features – Suggestive of Toxicity

• Vomiting and diarrhea (esp. ≤ 6h)	• Hypotension
• Mental status changes	• Coagulopathy, acidosis

Estimate of Quantity Elemental Iron Ingested and Toxicity Potential	Elemental Iron (page 100)	Toxicity
	< 20 mg/kg	None
	20-60 mg/kg	Mild to Moderate
	> 60 mg/kg	Severe

Serum Iron and TIBC levels

Obtain serum iron and total iron binding capacity (TIBC) at least 4 hours post-ingestion. Absorption and toxicity may be delayed for slow-release forms. Iron levels ≥ 350 µg/dl (normal 50-150) are serious, as the TIBC (350-500 µg/dl) may be exceeded. High iron falsely lowers TIBC measurements rendering this test unreliable.

Serum iron (µg/dl)	Toxicity
< 100	None
100-350	Mild
350-500	Moderate
500-1,000	Severe
> 1,000	Possibly lethal

Adjunctive Diagnostic Tests

WBC count	> 15,000 cells/mm^3 is associated with a serum iron > 300 µg/dl.
Glucose	> 150 g/dl is associated with a serum iron > 300 µg/dl.
KUB	Radio-opaque tablets on plain films indicate potential for further absorption/toxicity. 50% with iron > 300 µg/dl have negative X-ray.
Deferoxamine challenge	Test dose: 60-90 mg/kg IM. This agent binds free iron. After administration, pink or red urine indicates positive test. A negative test does **NOT** definitively exclude toxicity.

Treatment of Iron Poisoning

Fluid/blood	• Use NS ± blood prn. Consult surgeon if suspect perforation.
Decontaminate	• Lavage with NS (esp. if iron on xray). Charcoal is ineffective.
Whole bowel irrigation	• Administer polyethylene glycol (*GoLytely*). (page 95). This option is especially useful if Xray shows tablets beyond pylorus.
Deferoxamine	• 15 mg/kg/h IV infusion. Do not wait for iron levels to return if the patient is symptomatic. Deferoxamine given IV or IM causes↓ BP which is usually the limiting factor in infusion rate. Seizures can occur following deferoxamine. If improving, discontinue deferoxamine when urine clears and iron level <100 µg/dl.
Dialysis	• If renal failure prevents excretion of ferrioxamine

Indications for Chelation Therapy with Deferoxamine in Iron Toxicity	• Multisystem toxicity, eg, vomiting, diarrhea, GI bleeding, ↓BP, acidosis, altered mental status, coagulopathy
	• Tablets seen on plain abdominal radiograph
	• Positive deferoxamine challenge test
	• Serum iron > 350 µg/dl or serum iron greater than the TIBC (TIBC can be unreliable when serum iron levels are high)

Mushrooms

Treat all toxic mushroom ingestions with IV fluids and GI decontamination. Specific antidotes are useful for certain classes of mushrooms as discussed below. Toxic mushrooms in groups I, II and VIII cause delayed symptoms (>6h from ingestion).

	Phase	Time	Features
Phases of cyclopeptide mushroom toxicity	0	0-6h	asymptomatic latent phase (may last 24h)
	1	6-12h	gastrointestinal phase: vomiting, diarrhea
	2	12-24h	symptoms decrease, LFT's increase
	3	>24h	liver failure, shock, renal failure

Clinical Features, Onset, Treatment of Mushroom Toxicity

Group	Toxin	Onset	Symptoms	Treatment
I Cyclo-peptides	*cyclopeptides amatoxins phallatoxins virotoxins*	6-10h	See page 102	Multi-dose charcoal, IV NS, ± (penicillinG, cimetidine,thiotic acid, liver transplantation)
II MMH	*monomethyl-hydrazine (MMH)*	6-10h	CNS-seizures abdominal pain liver/renal failure	Pyridoxine ≥25 mg/kg IV, methylene blue for methemoglobinemia
III Muscarine	*muscarine*	½ - 2h	Cholinergic	Atropine
VI Coprine	*coprine*	½ - 2h	Disulfiram reaction (↑HR, flushed, vomit)	IV fluids
V Ibotinic acid and muscimol	*ibotenic acid, muscimol*	½ - 2h	GABA effects: (seizures, hal-ucinations), Anticholinergic	Benzodiazepines
VI Psilocybin	*psilocybin psilocin*	½ - 1h	Hallucinations (~LSD)	Benzodiazepines
VII GI toxins	*multiple*	½ - 3h	Pain, vomiting, diarrhea	IV fluids
VIII Orellines	*orelline, orellanine*	24 - 36h	Renal failure, vomiting	Supportive care, ± dialysis

Organophosphates and Carbamates

Organophosphates irreversibly bind and inhibit cholinesterases at CNS receptors, post-ganglionic parasympathetic nerves (muscarinic effects), and autonomic ganglia and skeletal myoneural junctions (nicotinic effects). Carbamates irreversibly bind cholinesterases and are less toxic.

Clinical Features of Insecticide Toxicity

Onset of symptoms	• Usually begin < 24h after exposure. Lipid-soluble organophos-phates (e.g. fenthion) may take days to produce symptoms with persistence for weeks to months and periodic relapses.
CNS	• Cholinergic excess: delirium, confusion, seizures, respiratory depression. Carbamates have less central effects.
Muscarinic	• SLUDGE (salivation, lacrimation, urination, defecation, GI upset, emesis), miosis, bronchoconstriction, bradycardia.
Nicotinic	• Fasciculations, muscle weakness, sympathetic ganglia stimulation (hypertension, tachycardia, pallor, rarely mydriasis)

Diagnostic Studies in Insecticide Poisoning

Labs	• ↑glucose, ↑K⁺, ↑WBC, ↑amylase, glycosuria, proteinuria
EKG	• Early - ↑ in sympathetic tone (tachycardia) • Later - extreme parasympathetic tone (sinus bradycardia, AV block, and ↑QT)
Serum *(pseudo)* RBC *(plasma)* Cholinesterase	• Serum levels are more sensitive but less specific than RBC • Plasma levels return to normal before RBC levels • Mild cases: levels are < 50% of normal • Severe cases: levels are < 10% of normal

Treatment

General	• Support airway, breathing and blood pressure. Respiratory depression is the most common cause of death. • Medical personnel should gown and glove if dermal exposure. • Wash toxin off patient if dermal exposure. • Administer charcoal if oral ingestion.
Atropine	• Competitively blocks acetylcholine (Ach) at muscarinic (not nicotinic) receptors. Atropine may reverse CNS effects. • <u>Dose</u>: ≥ 0.05 mg/kg q 5 min Mix 50 mg in 500 ml NS & titrate • <u>Goal</u>: titrate to mild anticholinergic signs (dry mouth, secretions) and not to pupil size or heart rate. • Treatment failure is most often due to not using enough atropine.
Pralidoxime (2-PAM)	• PAM has endogenous anticholinergic effects, while reversing nicotinic & central effects. It does not reverse carbamate toxicity. • <u>Dose</u>: 20-50 mg/kg IV over 15 minutes. May repeat q 10-12 hours. Onset of effect is 10-40 minutes after administration.
Atrovent	• Ipratropium bromide 0.5 mg nebulized q4-6h may dry secretions.

Salicylates

Methylsalicylate (oil of wintergreen) is the most toxic form. Absorption generally is within 1h of ingestion (delays ≥ 6h occur with enteric-coated and viscous preparations). At toxic levels, salicylates are renally metabolized. Alkaline urine promotes excretion. At different acidosis/alkalosis states, measurable salicylate levels change, therefore measure arterial pH at same time as drug level.

Ingestion	Severity	Signs and Symptoms
<150 mg/kg	mild	vomiting, tinnitus, and hyperpnea
150-300 mg/kg	moderate	vomiting, hyperpnea, diaphoresis, and tinnitus
>300 mg/kg	severe	acidosis, altered mental status, seizures, & shock

Clinical Features of Salicylate Toxicity

Direct	• Irritation of GI tract with reports of perforation
Metabolic	• <u>Early</u>: respiratory alkalosis from respiratory center stimulation. • <u>Later</u>: metabolic acidosis - uncoupled oxidative phosphorylation • Hypokalemia, ↑or↓ glucose, ketonuria, and either ↑or↓ Na+
CNS	• <u>Early</u>: tinnitus, deafness, agitation, hyperactivity • <u>Later</u>: confusion, lethargy, coma, seizure, CNS edema (esp. < 4y)
GI	• Vomiting, gastritis, pylorospasm, ↑ liver enzymes, perforation
Pulmonary	• Noncardiac pulmonary edema (esp. with chronic toxicity)

Indicators of Salicylate Toxicity

Clinical	• Features listed above are associated with toxicity
Ingestion	• Ingestion of ≥ 150 mg/kg is associated with toxicity
Ferric chloride	• Mix 2 drops $FeCl_3$+ 1 ml urine. Purple = salicylate ingestion
Phenstix	• Dipstick test for urine. Brown indicates salicylate or pheno-thiazine ingestion (not toxicity). Adding 1 drop 20N H_2SO_4 bleaches out color for phenothiazines but not salicylates.
Salicylate Levels	• A level > 30 mg/dl drawn ≥ 6h after ingestion is toxic. • Follow serial levels (q2-3h) until downward trend established. • Arterial pH must be measured at same time, as acidemia increases CNS penetration and toxicity at lower levels. • *Done nomogram has been proven unreliable.*
Nontoxic Ingestion	• If none of the following are present, acute toxicity is unlikely (1) < 150 mg/kg ingested, (2) absent clinical features (3) level < 30 mg/dl obtained ≥ 6h after ingestion (unless enteric coated preparation, viscous preparation, or chronic ingestion)

Treatment

General	• Treat dehydration, electrolyte abnormalities. CSF hypoglycemia occurs with normal serum glucose – add D_5 or D_{10} to all fluids.
Decontaminate	• Multi-dose charcoal. Whole bowel irrigation (if enteric coated).
Alkalinization	• Add 100 mEq $NaHCO_3$ to 1 L $D_5\frac{1}{2}$ NS (± 20-40 mEq/L K+ if no renal failure). <u>Goal</u> – urine pH > 7.5
Hemodialysis	• <u>Indications</u>: renal failure, noncardiogenic pulmonary edema, congestive heart failure, persistent CNS disturbances, deterioration of vital signs, unable to correct acid-base or electrolyte imbalance, salicylate level > 100 mg/dl (acutely)

Chronic Toxicity

Presentation	• Patients are generally older, on chronic salicylates. Neurologic changes and non-cardiogenic pulmonary edema are more common than with acute toxicity. Many are treated for infectious or neurologic disease prior to correct diagnosis.
Toxicity	• Salicylate levels are often normal to therapeutic.
Treatment	• Supportive measures & urinary alkalinization are recommended. Dialyze if acidosis, confusion, or pulmonary edema.

Theophylline
Clinical Features

Cardiovascular	• Tachycardia, atrial and ventricular dysrhythmias
Neurological	• Agitation, tremors, seizures
Metabolic	• ↑Glucose, ↑catecholamines, ↓potassium
Gastrointestinal	• Vomiting

Treatment

General	• Monitor for seizures, and arrhythmias. Correct dehydration, hypoxia, and electrolyte imbalances.
Charcoal	• Administer 1g/kg q2-4h. Repeat doses q4h.
Arrhythmias	• β-blockade is preferred for tachyarrhythmias (page 57). Do not use verapamil. It inhibits theophylline metabolism.
Seizures	• Use benzodiazepines (e.g. lorazepam) followed by barbiturates (e.g. phenobarbital). Phenytoin is *contraindicated*.
Hemoperfusion	• Indications (1) seizures, (2) poorly responsive arrhythmias, (3) theophylline level > 100 µg/ml in acute overdose or (4) theophylline level > 60 µg/ml in chronic overdose.

Tricyclic Antidepressants (TCA)

Clinical features are due to α adrenergic blockade (↓BP), anti-cholinergic effects (altered mentation, seizures, ↑HR, mydriasis), inhibition of norepinephrine uptake (increasing catecholamines) and Na+ channel blockade (causing quinidine like depressive effect on the heart). [1]ms – milliseconds; [2]bundle branch block	ECG findings in TCA overdose
	• Sinus tachycardia
	• ↑QRS > 100 ms[1], ↑PR interval, ↑QT interval, BBB[2] (esp. right BBB)
	• Right axis deviation of the terminal 40 ms of the QRS > 120 degrees
	• AV conduction blocks (all degrees)
	• Ventricular fibrillation or tachycardia (only occur in 4% who die from TCA's)

Treatment of TCA Toxicity

General	• Apply cardiac monitor, obtain baseline EKG to assess QRS width and QT interval
Decontamination	• Administer charcoal 1 g/kg PO or NG q2-4h. • Consider gastric lavage as anticholinergic effects may slow gastrointestinal transit. • Ensure patent airway & gag reflex prior to decontamination. • Avoid ipecac, as patients may have rapid mental status decline or develop seizures.
NaHCO₃	• <u>Indications</u>: (1) acidosis, (2) QRS width > 100 milliseconds, (3) ventricular arrhythmias, or (4) hypotension. • Alkalinization enhances TCA protein binding and reverses Na⁺ channel blockade and toxic cardiac manifestations. • <u>Dose</u>: 1-2 mEq/kg IV. • <u>Goal</u>: Arterial pH of 7.50-7.55. • NaHCO₃ is ineffective for CNS manifestations (e.g. seizures)
Fluids/pressors	• Administer 10-20 ml/kg NS for hypotension. Repeat 1-2 X. • If fluids are ineffective administer phenylephrine or norepinephrine (not dopamine) due pure α effects.
Anti-seizure medications	• Use lorazepam followed by phenobarbital. • Phenytoin may be ineffective in TCA-induced seizures.
MgSO₄	• 25 mg/kg administered slow IV (over 15 minutes) may be useful for ↓ BP, and arrhythmias.
Disposition	*Transfer to a psychiatric facility if all of the following are present:* • no major evidence of toxicity during 6h ED observation • active bowel sounds • ≥ 2 charcoal doses are given • there is no evidence of toxic coingestant.

Abuse and Neglect

Appearance of Cutaneous Bruises Over Time[1]	0 - 2 days	swollen, tender, red, blue, purple
	3 - 6 days	blue, green
	6 - 10 days	green, brown
	10 - 14 days	tan, yellow
	14 - 30 days	faded to clear

[1]Dating bruises based on color is not 100% accurate and ages are only a rough estimate.
Note: any bite marks with distance between incisors > 3 cm was made by an adult.

Bony Injuries Associated with Child Abuse

Fractures Associated With a High or Moderate Risk of Abuse	• Metaphyseal-epiphyseal fractures (e.g. corner, bucket handle, and metaphyseal lucency)
	• Posterior rib fractures
	• Fractures in different stages of healing
	• Fractures inconsistent with history or development of child
	• Avulsion fractures of the clavicle or acromion process
	• Skull – if multiple, depressed, or across suture line
	• Pelvic or spinal fractures without significant force
	• Spinous process, vertebral body fractures and subluxations
	• Femur fractures ≤ 1 year old
	• Fracture with delay in bringing child to the hospital
	• Scapular fractures
	• Sternal fractures
	• Non-supracondylar humerus fracture
Fractures Associated With a Low Risk of Abuse	• Clavicle fractures (except avulsion fractures)
	• Distal tibia spiral fractures (Toddler's fracture)
	• Supracondylar fractures
	• Fractures of the hand or feet
	• Torus fractures of long bones

Pediatr Emerg Med Reports 1998; 3: 1.

Components Of Skeletal Survey for Suspected Child Abuse	• Skull radiography (AP[1] & lateral views)
	• Chest radiography (AP[1] & lateral views)
	• Lateral spine radiography
	• Extremity AP[1] radiography
	• Pelvis AP[1] radiography

[1]AP – anterior-posterior film   *Emerg Med Reports* 1993; 14: 67

Trauma Scoring and Assessment

Pediatric Trauma Score[1]

Patient features	Score +2	Score +1	Score -1
Size (kg)	>20	10-20	<10
Airway	normal	maintainable	Non-maintainable
Systolic BP (mmHg)	>90	50-90	<50
Mental status	awake	obtunded	comatose
Open wound	none	minor	major
Extremity fractures	none	closed	open or multiple

[1]A total score of ≤ 8 suggests the need for a specialized trauma center. A score of < 1 predicts a mortality rate of >98%, a score of 4 predicts ~50% mortality, and a score of > 8 predicts < 1% mortality   *Ramnofsky: J Trauma 1988; 28:1038.*

Pediatric Glasgow Coma Scale[1]

Eye opening	Best motor	Best verbal
0-1 years 4. spontaneous 3. to shout 2. to pain 1. no response	**0-1 year** 6. spontaneous movement 5. localizes pain 4. flexion withdrawal 3. flexion / decorticate 2. extension / decerebrate 1. no response	**0-2 years** 5. normal cry, smile, coo 4. cries 3. inappropriate cry, scream 2. grunts 1. no response
>1 year 4. spontaneous 3. to verbal 2. to pain 1. no response	**>1 year** 6. obeys 5. localizes pain 4. flexion withdrawal 3. flexion / decorticate 2. extension / decerebrate 1. no response	**2-5 years** 5. appropriate words 4. inappropriate words 3. cries or screams 2. grunts 1. no response
		>5 years 5. oriented 4. disoriented but converses 3. inappropriate words 2. incomprehensible 1. no response

[1]Total score indicates that injury is mild (13-15), moderate (9-12), or severe (≤ 8).

Initial Approach to Pediatric Trauma

Primary Survey (0-5 minutes)	
Assessment	**Action**
Airway - assess air movement, while immobilizing cervical spine	Endotracheal intubate if (1) unable to ventilate, (2) altered mentation/aspiration risk, (3) need for hyperventilation in head injury, (4) flail chest, (5) severe shock See page 12 for ETT size and rapid sequence technique.
Breathing - assess ventilation effectiveness and oxygenation	Apply pulse oximeter (± end-tidal CO_2 monitor), O_2, perform needle thoracostomy for tension pneumothorax, occlusive dressing for sucking chest wound, and ETT if needed.
Circulation - assess strength, rate, quality of peripheral pulses, while stopping external bleed. See page 3 for complete list of normal vitals by age, weight, length. See pg 10 for central venous cath. sizes, and IO technique.	Attach cardiac monitor, apply pressure to external bleed, Assess peripheral pulse rate, quality, strength. Insert two large peripheral venous lines, and draw blood for type and crossmatch, and basic labs.

Age	IV catheter size	Intraosseous size
0-1 year	20-22 gauge	17 Fr
>1-6 years	18-20 gauge	15 Fr
8-12 years	16-20 gauge	-
> 15 years	14-18 gauge	-

Disability - assess pupils and alertness (AVPU)	Assess pupils + Peds Glasgow Coma scale (pg 109), AVPU (**A**lert, responds to **V**oice, **P**ain, **U**nresponsive)
Exposure	Completely undress patient (begin radiant warming)

Resuscitation (Simultaneously Performed during Primary Survey)	
Airway/Breathing	Reassess - see above
Circulation	Note: do not spend > 2-3 min attempting peripheral IV if hypotensive, obtain IO or central venous access. Administer NS 20 ml/kg IV for hypotension/shock. Reassess, and repeat NS 20 ml/kg IV if needed. Administer Oneg whole blood or packed RBC's 10-20 ml/kg. Insert NG tube, Foley catheter (see page 3 or 117 for size).

Secondary Survey and Definitive Care	
Reassess ABCDE	Address any deterioration or new abnormalities. Insert chest tube prn (e.g. if prior needle thoracostomy)
Head to toe examination	Complete vital signs (do not forget back and rectal exams).
Address extremity injuries	Reduce dislocations compromising circulation.
Initial Xrays	Obtain cervical spine, chest, pelvis, extremity, CT scans.
Pain control, infection risk	Administer analgesics, antibiotics, tetanus.
Begin disposition	Call surgeon, and consultants as need identified. Initiate transfer, admission, or prepare for operating room. Splint fractures and dress wounds.
Documentation	Document all abnormalities (including xray, lab abnormalities), consults and times. Talk to family.

Head and Neck Trauma

Management of Increased Intracranial Pressure following Trauma

- Perform rapid sequence intubation while immobilizing cervical spine (pg 12).
- Keep pO_2 at least 90 mm Hg and pCO_2 at 35 mm Hg. (pCO_2 25-30 if herniating)
- Maintain normal BP and keep head of bed 30-45 degrees(if no spine fracture).
- Minimize stimuli such as pain, suctioning and movement.
- Consider mannitol 0.25-1.0 g/kg IV + sedative if hemodynamically stable.
- Consider anti-seizure meds (fosphenytoinPE - 15-20mg/kg IV < 2mg/kg/min) if

Glasgow Coma Scale < 9	Subdural hematoma	Large contusion
Delayed seizure	Depressed fracture with parenchymal damage	

- Maintain ICP as close to normal (15-20 mm Hg) as possible.
  CPP (cerebral perfusion pressure) = MAP - ICP.

Risk Stratification and Imaging for Head Trauma

Low Risk	Moderate Risk	High Risk
Age > 2 years	Age < 2 unless trivial injury	Depressed level of cons-
Asymptomatic	Altered consciousness	ciousness (LOC) not
Headache alone	during or after event	clearly due to other
Dizziness	Multiple trauma	cause
Scalp hematoma	Progressive headache,vomiting	Focal neurologic signs
(except < 1-2 years)	Intoxication/unreliable history	Decreasing LOC
Scalp contusion, abrasion	Post trauma seizure	Penetrating skull injury or
Absence of moderate	Basilar skull fracture signs, pos	palpable skull depression
and high risk criteria	sible skull depression or pen-	
	etration, or Suspected abuse	
Recommendation	*Recommendation*	*Recommendation*
Observation, with head	Extended close observation	CT scan and neurosurgical
injury instructions	CT scan with possible	consultation
(To date: studies attempting	neurosurgical consultation	
to identify high or low yield	Skull films - rarely indicated	
indications for cranial CT	unless looking for old abuse,	Masters *New Engl J Med*
have been unsuccessful)	growing fracture	1987; 316: 85.

Criteria for Cervical Spine Imaging in Blunt Trauma

Neck pain, not confined to trapezius	Severe traumatic mechanism
Impaired consciousness, poor history	• fall from height
Motor or sensory complaints or deficits	• pedestrian hit by car
Multi-system trauma	• diving injury
Distracting injury or pain	Trauma with underlying spine instability
Prior cervical spine fracture or surgery	• Down's, JRA, Klippel-Feil syndrome

Normal Cervical Spine spaces

A - Predental space < 5mm if < 8 years old, otherwise < 3 mm.

B - Posterior cervical line, spino-laminar line of C2 should be within 2 mm anterior or posterior to this line.

C - Prevertebral space ≤ 7 mm in front of C2 or < 1/3 of width of C2 vertebral body.

D - Limit of overriding of vertebral bodies is 2.5 mm.

E - Retrotracheal space should be < 14 mm in front of C6 or < 5/4 of width of C5 in front of C5.

F - Prevertebral fat stripe - should not bulge out.

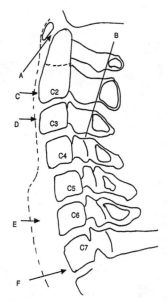

Used with permission – *Pediatr Emerg Med Reports* 1996;1:83.

Cervical Spine Anatomy in Children < 8 years old
Normal lordosis to cervical spine is absent in 14% of children
Majority of injuries occur at C1-C2 ≤ 8 years old and lower cervical spine > 8 years
Os odontoideum - congenital anomaly where odontoid does not fuse with C2[a]
Ossiculum terminale - congenital failure of dens apex fusion by age 12-14
Prevertebral space at C3 is ≤1/3-2/3 of C3 vertebral body width or ≤ 5-7 mm[b]
Prevertebral space at C5 is ≤ 5/4 of C5 vertebral body width or ≤ 14 mm[b]
Predental space up to 5 mm ≤ 8 years (up to 3 mm > 8 years)
Pseudo-Jeffersonian fx-C1 lateral masses grow faster than C2 so C1 overlaps C2
Pseudosubluxation of C2/C3 or C3/C4 in 40% (normal variant where anterior aspect
of C2 spinolaminar line is ≤ 2 mm ant or post to posterior cervical line(B on pg 112)

[a]spine injury with minor trauma occurs, [b] these norms can be unreliable in children

Development of Cervical Spine

Age	Feature
< 6 mo	C1 ring invisible and all synchondroses are open, vertebrate are normally wedged anteriorly, and there is often no lordosis to the un-injured spine
1 yr	body of C1 becomes visible radiographically
3 yr	posteriorly located spinous process synchondroses fuse
	dens becomes ossified (visible radiographically)
3-6 yr	neurocentral (body) and C2-odontoid synchondroses fuse
	summit ossification center appears at the apex (top) of the odontoid
	anterior wedging of the vertebral bodies resolve (and is normal if seen)
8 yr	pseudosubluxation and predental widening resolve, lordosis is normal now
12-14	secondary ossification centers appear at spinous process tips (often mistaken for fractures), summit ossification center of odontoid fuses (if it does not *os odontoideum* occurs), superior/inferior epiphyseal rings appear on body
25 yr	secondary ossification centers at tips of spinous processes fuse
	superior/inferior epiphyseal rings fuse to vertebral body

Spinal Cord Injury without Radiologic Abnormality (SCIWORA)

SCIWORA accounts for 1/5 of all pediatric spinal cord injuries. Immediate plain films, CT and MRI are normal with atrophy of spinal cord evident on MRI performed 1-3 mo after accident. 54% have a delayed onset of neurologic deficit (mean 1.2 days) with half of the delayed subset complaining of paresthesias at the time of the accident.   83% involve the cervical cord, and 2/3 are ≤ 8 years old. For children with delayed paralysis, progression of weakness is rapid and usually causes complete cord lesion.

Spinal Cord Injury Syndromes[1, 2]

Anterior Cord Syndrome	Central Cord Syndrome
• Flexion or vertical compression injury to anterior cord or spinal artery • Complete motor paralysis • Hyperalgesia with preserved touch and proprioception (position sense) • Loss of pain and temperature sense • Most likely cord injury to require surgery	• Hyperextension injury • Motor weakness in hands > arms • Legs are unaffected or less affected • Variable bladder/sensory dysfunction • Prognosis is generally good and most do not require surgery
Complete Cord Injury	**Brown-Sequard Syndrome**
• Flaccid below injury level • Absent deep tendon reflexes • Decreased sympathetics • Warm skin, low BP, and slow HR • Sensation may be preserved • Priapism may be present • If lasts > 24 hours, will be complete	• Hemisection of cord • Ipsilateral weakness • Ipsilateral loss of proprioception • Contralateral loss of pain and temperature sensation
	Posterior Cord Syndrome
	• Pain, tingling, of neck and hands • 1/3 have upper extremity weakness • Mild form of central cord syndrome

[1] diffuse flexion withdrawal movements can occur in children with paralyzed limbs in response to stimulation mimicking normal movements.

[2] see page 126 for dermatomes, muscles, and reflexes.

Steroid Protocol for Treatment of Acute Spinal Cord Injury

- *Indications*: Acute spinal cord injury presenting within **8 hours** of injury.
- *Contraindications* (absolute and relative): Age < 13 years (controversial), nerve root or cauda equina syndrome, gun shot wounds, pregnancy, already on steroids, and other life threatening illness.
- *Protocol*: methylprednisolone 30 mg/kg IV over 15 minutes, followed by 45 min pause, followed by methylprednisolone 5.4 mg/kg/hour IV (1) over 23 hours if < 3 hours since injury and (2) over 47 hours if 3-8 hours since injury.

Bracken *New Engl J Med* 1990; 322: 1405; Bracken *JAMA* 1997; 277: 1597.

Thoracic Trauma

Differentiating between Immediate Life Threatening Thoracic Injuries

Feature	Tension pneumothorax	Massive hemothorax	Cardiac tamponade
breath sounds	ipsilateral diminished	ipsilateral diminished	equal
percussion	hyperresonant	dull	equal
trachea	shifted away from tension	midline	midline
neck veins[1]	distended	normal or flat	distended
heart tones	normal	normal	diminished

[1] unreliable as neck veins may be flat due to hypovolemia in all cases.

Other Serious Thoracic Injuries

Injury	Clinical Features, Diagnosis, Management
Diaphragmatic rupture	Due to $\uparrow$ abdominal pressures (left > right sided). Abdominal contents herniate into chest. CXR may show $\uparrow$ diaphragm, gastric dilation, subpulmonic hemopneumothroax, or NG in chest. Treat by placing NG, ETT, and surgery.
Esophageal rupture	Extremely rare injury. Chest tube drain of apparent hemothorax reveals food, saliva, or bubbles with respiration. Treat surgically.
Flail chest	Double fractures of 2 adjacent ribs with paradoxic inspiratory collapse, + expiratory bulge of lung. Often pulmonary contusion exist. Intubate, use positive pressure ventilation, PEEP, and paralyze.
Myocardial contusion	Extremely rare in children. EKG, cardiac enzymes, and echocardiogram are insensitive. Children generally need monitoring.
Open Pneumothorax (Sucking chest wound)	Loss of chest wall equal or greater than the size of a bronchus. Paradoxic ventilation with to and fro movement of the mediastinum so both lungs collapse on inspiration. Cover 3 sides of defect with sterile dressing. After chest tube placed, cover defect with airtight dressing.
Pulmonary contusion	Early CXR and exam may be relatively normal. Treat supportively. Consider ETT + PEEP (5-10 cm) if $pO_2 < 70mmHg$, despite FiO_2 40%.
Rib fracture	Uncommon. Posterior fracture may indicate abuse. No treatment.
Hemothorax	Need up to 10ml/kg of blood to show up on CXR. Place chest tube.
Pneumothorax	If multiple trauma, chest tube is always indicated. (see below)
Thoracic aorta rupture	CXR may show wide mediastinum, trachea or NG deviated to right, 1st or 2nd rib fracture, or apical pleural cap. Treat surgically.
Traumatic asphyxia	Due to a sudden $\uparrow$ in thoracic pressure transmitted to head, neck, and torso veins. CNS bleeding can occur. Treatment is supportive.

Chest tube sizes (French) for Traumatic Hemothorax/Pneumothorax

Age (years)	1mo	0.5	1	3	5-6	8	12	16
Size	12-18	14-20	14-24	16-28	20-32	24-32	28-36	28-40

Emerg Med Clin North Am 1993; 11: 187.

Abdominal Trauma

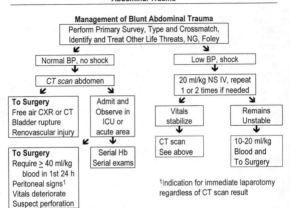

Management of Blunt Abdominal Trauma

Perform Primary Survey, Type and Crossmatch,
Identify and Treat Other Life Threats, NG, Foley

Normal BP, no shock → *CT scan* abdomen

To Surgery
Free air CXR or CT
Bladder rupture
Renovascular injury

Admit and Observe in ICU or acute area

To Surgery
Require ≥ 40 ml/kg blood in 1st 24 h
Peritoneal signs[1]
Vitals deteriorate
Suspect perforation

Serial Hb
Serial exams

Low BP, shock → 20 ml/kg NS IV, repeat 1 or 2 times if needed

Vitals stabilize → CT scan See above

Remains Unstable → 10-20 ml/kg Blood and To Surgery

[1]Indication for immediate laparotomy regardless of CT scan result

CT vs. US vs. Diagnostic Peritoneal Lavage (DPL) in Blunt Abdominal Trauma

	Computed Tomography (CT)[1]	DPL	Ultrasound (US)
Main Indication	(1)Stable vitals, + blunt trauma, altered mental status, CNS pelvic, spine, or significant thoracic trauma, or hematuria. (2) Unexplained hypotension, or dropping hemoglobin *Reuss AJR 1997;169: 1011*	Unstable with other need for an operation (e.g.CNS trauma) *Powell J Trauma 1987;27: 6.*	Immediate bedside assessment for peritoneal blood. *Katz J Pediatr Surg 1996;649.*
Advantage	More than 95% sensitivity for laparotomy need, major vascular, solid organ, significant retroperitoneal injury	Nearly 99% sensitive in diagnosis of surgical injury	Detects blood in > 90 to 95% requiring laparotomy for blunt abdominal trauma
Drawback	May miss hollow organ injury, pancreas injury, minor renal (esp. ureteral) injury, mesenteric or diaphragm injury	Does not tell specific organ injured, many false positives	Poor at identifying specific organ injured.

[1]recent studies indicate oral contrast may be unnecessary for CT in acute trauma.

Renal and Genitourinary Trauma

Diagnostic Evaluation of Suspected Blunt Renal Trauma

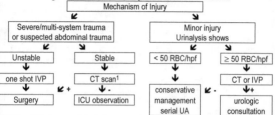

[1]CT-if multiple trauma, abdominal trauma, shock, pelvic, lumbar, thoracic or lower rib fracture. CT or IVP if minor trauma, or suspected ureteral injury (e.g. penetrating trauma). *Morey J Urol 1996; 156: 2014.*

Evaluation of Suspected Urethral Trauma

Retrograde Urethrogram Indications	Retrograde Urethrogram Technique
Penile, perineal, vaginal or scrotal trauma	Obtain preinjection KUB film
Blood at urethral meatus or cannot void	Place Cooke adapter or Christmas tree
Extravasation of blood/urine to scrotum, perineum, abdominal wall or penile shaft	adapter on end of 30-60 ml syringe. (may substitute Foley - see below)
Abnormal prostate examination	Inject 0.2 ml/kg of contrast dye over 60
Significant pelvic fracture	seconds
Inability to easily pass Foley catheter	Take xray during last 10 seconds

Evaluation of Suspected Bladder Trauma

Cystogram Indications	Cystogram Technique
Penetrating injury to low abdomen or pelvis	After urethrogram empty bladder
Blunt lower abdominal-perineal trauma with significant microscopic hematuria (> 20 RBC/ hpf), gross blood, blood at meatus	Instill contrast into bladder using 5ml/kg or discomfort or bladder is full (see formula below for normal bladder volumes)
Significant pelvic fracture	Obtain oblique, and AP films of bladder,
Unable to void or minimal urine after Foley	empty bladder then repeat films.

Bladder volume if [< 1 yr = weight (kg) X 10 ml]; if [≥ 1 yr =(age in years + 2) x 30 ml]

Estimated Urethral Catheter Size (French) Based on Age (Years)

Age	1 day	3 mo	1	3	6	8	10	12	teen
Size	5	8	8-10	10	10	10-12	12	12-14	16+

Genital Disorders - Male

The Painful Scrotum

Feature	Torsion of Testicle	Epididymitis & Orchitis	Torsion of Testicular Appendix
Frequency, age 0-20 yr	25-50%	10-25%	30-50%
Frequency, age 20-29	20%	80%	0%
Pain onset	acute onset	gradual onset	gradual onset
Pain location	testis, groin, abdomen	testes, groin, epididymis	testis or upper pole
Prior similar episodes	often	rare	rare
Fever	rare	up to 1/3	rare
Dysuria	rare	common	rare
Testicle/Scrotum	horizontal high riding testis	firm, red, warm scrotum (>70%)	usually nontender, blue-dot upper testis
Cremasteric reflex	usually absent	may be present	may be present
Pyuria	up to 10%	25-60%	rare
Doppler / Nuclear scan	↓ flow	↑ flow	normal flow

Evaluation

- Contact urologist immediately if torsion suspected. Immediate surgical exploration has best chance of saving testicle. If clinical suspicion is low, consider one of diagnostic tests below after consultation with urologist.
- Doppler has 80-90% sensitivity and specificity in diagnosing testicular torsion. Absent flow is suspicious for torsion while intact flow suggests inflammation. Perform funicular compression during Doppler: Compress the testicular artery to see if flow stops. This signifies observed Doppler flow was testicular, not scrotal.
- Nuclear scan is ~85% sensitive & > 95% specific for torsion. False negative exams occur if small testicles (infants), spontaneous detorsion, or early torsion.
- Color Doppler flow is 86-100% sensitive and 100% specific for torsion in adults.

Pediatr Clin North Am 1997; 44: 1065.

	Knight and Vassey Criteria
If ≥ 3 of the 6 *Knight and Vassey* criteria were present, risk of testicular torsion risk was 0% in Knight & Vassey's study. In this study, no torsion cases occurred in 395 children who had ≥ 3 criteria, while all 130 confirmed testicular torsion cases had < 3 criteria. Furthermore, the presence of a *cremasteric reflex* almost always excludes torsion, although its absence is not specific for any disorder.	• Gradual pain onset • Dysuria, urethral discharge, recent cystocopy, or indwelling Foley • History of UTI, imperforate anus, hypospadias, or bladder dysfunction • Temperature > 101 F • Tender/indurated epididymis • > 10 WBC/high power field in urine Knight, Vassey. *Ann Surg* 1984; 200: 664

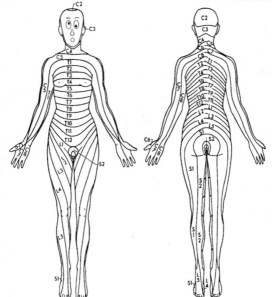

Motor level	Motor function
C4	spontaneous breathing
C5	shoulder shrug
C6	elbow flexion
C7	elbow extension
C8/T1	finger flexion
T1-T12	intercostal and abdominal muscles

Motor level	Motor function
L1/L2	hip flexion
L3	hip adduction
L4	hip abduction
L5	great toe dorsiflexion
S1/S2	foot plantar flexion
S2-S4	rectal tone